Environmental Health Criteria 118

INORGANIC MERCURY

Published under the joint sponsorship of
the United Nations Environment Programme,
the International Labour Organisation,
and the World Health Organization

First draft prepared by Dr L. Friberg,
Karolinska Institute, Sweden

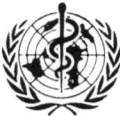

World Health Organization
Geneva, 1991

The **International Programme on Chemical Safety (IPCS)** is a joint venture of the United Nations Environment Programme, the International Labour Organisation, and the World Health Organization. The main objective of the IPCS is to carry out and disseminate evaluations of the effects of chemicals on human health and the quality of the environment. Supporting activities include the development of epidemiological, experimental laboratory, and risk-assessment methods that could produce internationally comparable results, and the development of manpower in the field of toxicology. Other activities carried out by the IPCS include the development of know-how for coping with chemical accidents, coordination of laboratory testing and epidemiological studies, and promotion of research on the mechanisms of the biological action of chemicals.

WHO Library Cataloguing in Publication Data

Inorganic mercury.

(Environmental health criteria ; 118)

1.Mercury poisoning   2.Environmental pollutants   I.Series

ISBN 92 4 157118 7   (NLM Classification: QV 293)
ISSN 0250-863X

CONTENTS

ENVIRONMENTAL HEALTH CRITERIA FOR
INORGANIC MERCURY

WHO TASK GROUP ON ENVIRONMENTAL HEALTH CRITERIA FOR INORGANIC MERCURY

Members

Professor M. Berlin, Institute of Environmental Medicine, University of Lund, Lund, Sweden (*Chairman*)

Professor P. Druet, Broussais Hospital, Paris, France

Professor V. Foà, Institute of Occupational Health, University of Milan, Milan, Italy

Professor L. Friberg, Karolinska Institute, Department of Environmental Hygiene, Stockholm, Sweden

Professor P. Glantz, Prosthetic Dentistry, Faculty of Odontology, University of Lund, Tandlakarhogskolan, Malmö, Sweden

Professor C.A. Gotelli, Centre for Toxicological Research, Buenos Aires, Argentina

Professor G. Kazantzis, Institute of Occupational Health, London School of Hygiene and Tropical Medicine, London, United Kingdom (*Rapporteur*)

Dr L. Magos, Toxicological Unit, Medical Research Council, Carshalton, Surrey, United Kingdom

Dr W.B. Peirano, Environmental Criteria and Assessment Office, Office of Research and Development, US Environmental Protection Agency, Cincinnati, USA

Professor B.S. Sridhara Rama Rao, Department of Neurochemistry, National Institute of Mental Health and Neurosciences, Bangalore, India

Professor M. Riolfatti, Institute of Hygiene, Faculty of Pharmaceutical Science, Padova, Italy

Dr M.J. Vimy, Health Science Centre, Department of Medicine and Medical Physiology, Faculty of Medicine, University of Calgary, Calgary, Alberta, Canada

Observers

Dr M. Ancora, Centro Italiano Studi e Indagini, Rome,
Italy

Professor K.S. Larsson, Institute for Odontological Toxicology, Faculty of Dentistry, Karolinska Institute,
Huddinge, Sweden

Professor C. Maltoni, Institute of Oncology, Bologna,
Italy

Dr A. Mochi, Centro Italiano Studi e Indagini, Rome, Italy

Professor A.A.G. Tomlinson, Centro Italiano Studi e
Indagini, Rome, Italy

Secretariat

Dr D. Kello, Toxicology and Food Safety, World Health
Organization Regional Office for Europe, Copenhagen,
Denmark

Dr T. Kjellström, Prevention of Environmental Pollution,
Division of Environmental Health, World Health Organization, Geneva, Switzerland (*Secretary*)

NOTE TO READERS OF THE CRITERIA MONOGRAPHS

Every effort has been made to present information in the criteria monographs as accurately as possible without unduly delaying their publication. In the interest of all users of the environmental health criteria monographs, readers are kindly requested to communicate any errors that may have occurred to the Manager of the International Programme on Chemical Safety, World Health Organization, Geneva, Switzerland, in order that they may be included in corrigenda, which will appear in subsequent volumes.

*   *   *

A detailed data profile and a legal file can be obtained from the International Register of Potentially Toxic Chemicals, Palais des Nations, 1211 Geneva 10, Switzerland (Telephone No. 7988400 or 7985850).

ENVIRONMENTAL HEALTH CRITERIA FOR INORGANIC MERCURY

A WHO Task Group on Environmental Health Criteria for Inorganic Mercury met in Bologna, Italy, at the County Council Headquarters (Provincia) from 25 to 30 September 1989. The meeting was sponsored by the Italian Ministry of the Environment and organized locally by the Institute of Oncology and Environmental Sciences with the assistance of the County Council. Professor C. Maltoni, Director of the Bologna Institute of Oncology, opened the meeting and welcomed the participants on behalf of the host institution. Mr A. Vecchi, Dr M. Moruzzi, and Dr A. Lolli, welcomed the participants on behalf of the local authorities. Dr A. Mochi, Centro Italiano Studi e Indagini, greeted the participants on behalf of the Ministry of the Environment, and Dr D. Kello, WHO Regional Office for Europe, addressed the meeting on behalf of the cooperating organizations of the IPCS (ILO/UNEP/WHO).

The Task Group reviewed and revised the draft document and made an evaluation of the human health risks from exposure to inorganic mercury.

The draft of this report was prepared by Dr L. Friberg, Karolinska Institute, Stockholm, Sweden. Dr T. Kjellström, WHO, Geneva, was responsible for the overall scientific content and Dr P.G. Jenkins, WHO, Geneva, for the technical editing.

*   *   *

Partial financial support for the publication of this report was kindly provided by the National Institute of Environmental Medicine, Stockholm, Sweden, and the Ministry of the Environment of Italy. The Centro Italiano Studi e Indagini and the Institute of Oncology, Bologna, contributed to the organization and provision of meeting facilities.

ABBREVIATIONS

AAS	atomic absorption spectrophotometry
CNS	central nervous system
CVAA	cold vapour atomic absorption
EEC	European Economic Community
EEG	electroencephalogram
GBM	glomerular basement membrane
GC	gas chromatography
GEMS	Global Environment Monitoring System
GLC	gas-liquid chromatography
LOAEL	lowest-observed-adverse-effect level
MGP	membranous glomerulopathy
NOAEL	no-observed-adverse-effect level
SD	standard deviation
SMR	standardized mortality ratio
TWA	time-weighted average

1. SUMMARY AND CONCLUSIONS

This monograph concentrates primarily on the risk to human health from inorganic mercury, and examines research reports that have appeared since the publication of Environmental Health Criteria 1: Mercury (WHO, 1976). In the period since 1976, new research data has become available for two main health concerns related to inorganic mercury, i.e. mercury in dental amalgam and in skin-lightening soaps. The emphasis in this monograph is on exposure from these two sources, but the basic kinetics and toxicology are reviewed with all aspects of inorganic mercury in mind.

Human health concerns related to the global transport, bioaccumulation, and transformation of inorganic mercury almost exclusively arise from the conversion of mercury compounds into methylmercury and exposure to methylmercury in sea-food and other food. The global environmental and ecological aspects of inorganic mercury have been summarized in this monograph. More detailed descriptions may be found in Environmental Health Criteria 86: Mercury - Environmental Aspects (WHO, 1989) and Environmental Health Criteria 101: Methylmercury (WHO, 1990).

1.1 Identity

Mercury exists in three states: Hg^0 (metallic); Hg_2^{++} (mercurous); and Hg^{++} (mercuric). It can form organometallic compounds, some of which have found industrial and agricultural uses.

1.2 Physical and chemical properties

Elemental mercury has a very high vapour pressure. The saturated atmosphere at 20 °C has a concentration over 200 times greater than the currently accepted concentration for occupational exposure.

Solubility in water increases in the order: elemental mercury < mercurous chloride < methylmercury chloride < mercuric chloride. Elemental mercury and the halide compounds of alkylmercurials are soluble in non-polar solvents.

Mercury vapour is more soluble in plasma, whole blood, and haemoglobin than in distilled water, where it dissolves only slightly. The organometallic compounds are stable, although some are readily broken down by living organisms.

1.3 Analytical methods

The most commonly used analytical methods for the quantification of total and inorganic mercury compounds are atomic absorption of cold vapour (CVAA) and neutron activation. Detailed information relating to analytical methods are given in Environmental Health Criteria 1: Mercury (WHO, 1976) and Environmental Health Criteria 101: Methylmercury (WHO, 1990).

All analytical procedures for mercury require careful quality control and quality assurance.

1.3.1 Analysis, sampling, and storage of urine

Flameless atomic absorption spectrophotometry is used in routine analysis for various media. Particular care must be taken when choosing the anticoagulant used for blood sampling in order to avoid contamination by mercury compounds. Special care must also be taken in the sampling and storage of urine, since bacterial growth can change the concentration of the numerous forms of mercury that may be present. Addition of hydrochloric acid or bactericidal substances and freezing the sample are the best methods to prevent alteration of urine samples. Correction of concentration by reference to urine density or creatinine content are recommended.

1.3.2 Analysis and sampling of air

Analytical methods for mercury in air may be divided into instant reading methods and methods with separate sampling and analysis stages. Instant reading methods can be used for the quantification of elemental mercury vapour. Sampling in acid-oxidizing media or on hopcalite is used for the quantification of total mercury.

The cold vapour atomic absorption (CVAA) technique is the most frequently used analytical method.

1.4 Sources of human and environmental exposure

1.4.1 Natural occurrence

The major natural sources of mercury are degassing of the earth's crust, emissions from volcanoes, and evaporation from natural bodies of water.

The natural emissions are of the order of 2700-6000 tonnes per year.

1.4.2 Sources due to human activities

The world-wide mining of mercury is estimated to yield about 10 000 tonnes/year. These activities lead to some losses of mercury and direct discharges to the atmosphere. Other important sources are fossil fuel combustion, metal sulfide ore smelting, gold refining, cement production, refuse incineration, and industrial applications of metals.

The specific normal emission from a chloralkali plant is about 450 g of mercury per ton of caustic soda produced.

The total global amount and release of mercury, due to human activities, to the atmosphere has been estimated to be up to 3000 tonnes/year.

1.5 Uses

A major use of mercury is as a cathode in the electrolysis of sodium chloride. Since the resultant chemicals are contaminated with mercury, their use in other industrial activities leads to a contamination of other products. Mercury is used in the electrical industry, in control instruments in the home and industry, and in laboratory and medical instruments. Some therapeutic agents contain inorganic mercury. A very large amount of mercury is used for the extraction of gold.

Dental silver amalgam for tooth filling contains large amounts of mercury, mixed (in the proportion of 1:1) with alloy powder (silver, tin, copper, zinc). Copper amalgam, used mostly in paediatric dentistry, contains up to 70%

mercury and up to 30% copper. These uses can cause exposure of the dentist, dental assistants, and also of the patients.

Some dark-skinned people use mercury-containing creams and soap to achieve a lighter skin tone. The distribution of these products is now banned in the EEC, in North America, and in many African countries, but mercury-containing soap is still manufactured in several European countries. The soaps contain up to 3% of mercuric iodine and the creams contain ammoniated mercury (up to 10%).

1.6 Environmental transport, distribution, and transformation

Emitted mercury vapour is converted to soluble forms and deposited by rain onto soil and water. The atmospheric residence time for mercury vapour is up to 3 years, whereas soluble forms have a residence time of only a few weeks.

The change in speciation of mercury from inorganic to methylated forms is the first step in the aquatic bioaccumulation process. This can occur non-enzymically or through microbial action. Methylmercury enters the foodchain of predatory species where biomagnification occurs.

1.7 Human exposure

The general population is primarily exposed to mercury through the diet and dental amalgam. Depending on the concentrations in air and water, significant contributions to the daily intake of total mercury can occur. Fish is a dominant source of human exposure to methylmercury. Recent experimental studies have shown that mercury is released from amalgam restorations in the mouth as vapour. The release rate of this mercury vapour is increased, for example, by chewing. Several studies have correlated the number of dental amalgam fillings or amalgam surfaces with the mercury content in tissues from human autopsy, as well as in samples of blood, urine, and plasma. Both the predicted mercury uptake from amalgam and the observed accumulation of mercury show substantial individual variation. It is, therefore, difficult to make accurate quantitative estimations of the mercury release and uptake by the human body from dental amalgam tooth restorations.

Experimental studies in sheep have examined in greater detail the distribution of mercury released from amalgam restorations.

Use of skin-lightening soap and creams can give rise to substantial mercury exposure.

Occupational exposure to inorganic mercury has been investigated in chloralkali plants, mercury mines, thermometer factories, refineries, and in dental clinics. High mercury levels have been reported for all these occupational exposure situations, although levels vary according to work environment conditions.

1.8 Kinetics and metabolism

Results of both human and animal studies indicate that about 80% of inhaled metallic mercury vapour is retained by the body, whereas liquid metallic mercury is poorly absorbed via the gastrointestinal tract (less than 1%). Inhaled inorganic mercury aerosols are deposited in the respiratory tract and absorbed, the rate depending on particle size. Inorganic mercury compounds are probably absorbed from the human gastrointestinal tract to a level of less than 10% on average, but there is considerable individual variation. Absorption is much higher in newborn rats.

The kidney is the main depository of mercury after the administration of elemental mercury vapour or inorganic mercury compounds (50-90% of the body burden of animals). Significantly more mercury is transported to the brain of mice and monkeys after the inhalation of elemental mercury than after the intravenous injection of equivalent doses of the mercuric form. The red blood cell to plasma ratio in humans is higher ($\geq$ 1) after administration of elemental mercury than mercuric mercury and more mercury crosses the placental barrier. Only a small fraction of the administered divalent mercury enters the rat fetus.

Several forms of metabolic transformation can occur:

- oxidation of metallic mercury to divalent mercury;
- reduction of divalent mercury to metallic mercury;
- methylation of inorganic mercury;

• conversion of methylmercury to divalent inorganic mercury.

The oxidation of metallic mercury vapour to divalent ionic mercury (section 6.1.1) is not fast enough to prevent the passage of elemental mercury through the blood-brain barrier, the placenta, and other tissues. Oxidation in these tissues serves as a trap to hold the mercury and leads to accumulation in brain and fetal tissues.

The reduction of divalent mercury to Hg^0 has been demonstrated both in animals (mice and rats) and humans. The decomposition of organomercurials, including methylmercury, is also a source of mercuric mercury.

The faecal and urinary routes are the main pathways for the elimination of inorganic mercury in humans, although some elemental mercury is exhaled. One form of depletion is the transfer of maternal mercury to the fetus.

The biological half-time, which only lasts a few days or weeks for most of the absorbed mercury, is very long, probably years, for a fraction of the mercury. Such long half-times have been observed in animal experiments as well as in humans. A complicated interplay exists between mercury and some other elements, including selenium. The formation of a selenium complex may be responsible for the long half-time of a fraction of the mercury.

1.8.1 Reference and normal values

Limited information from deceased miners shows mercury concentrations in the brain, years after cessation of exposure, of several mg/kg, with still higher values in some parts of the brain. However, lack of quality control of the analysis makes these data uncertain. Among a small number of deceased dentists, without known symptoms of mercury intoxication, mercury levels varied from very low concentrations up to a few hundred $\mu g/kg$ in the occipital lobe cortex and from about 100 $\mu g/kg$ to a few mg/kg in the pituitary gland.

From autopsies on subjects not occupationally exposed but with a varying number of amalgam fillings, it seems that a moderate number (about 25) of amalgam surfaces may on average increase the brain mercury concentration by about 10 μg/kg. The corresponding increase in the kidneys, based on a very limited number of analyses, is probably 300-400 μg/kg. However, the individual variation is considerable.

Mercury levels in urine and blood can be used as indicators of exposure provided that the exposure is recent and relatively constant, is long-term, and is evaluated on a group basis. Recent exposure data are more reliable than those quoted in Environmental Health Criteria 1: Mercury (WHO, 1976). Urinary levels of about 50 μg per g creatinine are seen after occupational exposure to about 40 μg mercury/m^3 of air. This relationship (5:4) between urine and air levels is much lower that the 3:1 estimated by WHO (1976). The difference may in part be explained by different sampling technique for evaluating air exposure. An exposure of 40 μg mercury/m^3 of air will correspond to about 15-20 μg mercury/litre of blood. However, interference from methylmercury exposure can make it difficult to evaluate exposure to low concentrations of inorganic mercury by means of blood analysis. A way to overcome the problems is to analyse mercury in plasma or analyse both inorganic mercury and methylmercury. The problem of interference from methylmercury is much smaller when analysing urine, as methylmercury is excreted in the urine to only a very limited extent.

1.9 Effects in humans

Acute inhalation exposure to mercury vapour may be followed by chest pains, dyspnoea, coughing, haemoptysis, and sometimes interstitial pneumonitis leading to death. The ingestion of mercuric compounds, in particular mercuric chloride, has caused ulcerative gastroenteritis and acute tubular necrosis causing death from anuria where dialysis was not available.

The central nervous system is the critical organ for mercury vapour exposure. Subacute exposure has given rise to psychotic reactions characterized by delirium, hallucinations, and suicidal tendency. Occupational exposure has resulted in erethism as the principal feature of a broad ranging functional disturbance. With continuing exposure a fine tremor develops, initially involving the hands. In the milder cases erethism and tremor regress slowly over a period of years following removal from exposure. Decreased nerve conduction velocity has been demonstrated in mercury-exposed workers. Long-term, low-level exposure has been associated with less pronounced symptoms of erethism.

There is very little information available on brain mercury levels in cases of mercury poisoning, and nothing that makes it possible to estimate a no-observed-effect level or a dose-response curve.

At a urinary mercury excretion level of 100 μg per g creatinine, the probability of developing the classical neurological signs of mercurial intoxication (tremor, erethism) and proteinuria is high. An exposure corresponding to 30 to 100 μg mercury/g creatinine increases the incidence of some less severe toxic effects that do not lead to overt clinical impairment. In a few studies tremor, recorded electrophysiologically, has been observed at low urine concentrations (down to 25-35 μg/g creatinine). Other studies did not show such an effect. Some of the exposed people develop proteinuria (proteins of low relative molecular mass and microalbuminuria). Appropriate epidemiological data covering exposure levels corresponding to less than 30-50 μg mercury/g creatinine are not available.

The exposure of the general population is generally low, but may occasionally be raised to the level of occupational exposure and can even be toxic. Thus, the mishandling of liquid mercury has resulted in severe intoxication.

The kidney is the critical organ following the ingestion of inorganic divalent mercury salts. Occupational exposure to metallic mercury has long been associated with the development of proteinuria, both in workers with other evidence of mercury poisoning and in those without such evidence. Less commonly, occupational exposure has been followed by the nephrotic syndrome, which has also occurred after the use of skin-lightening creams containing inorganic mercury, and even after accidental exposure. The current evidence suggests that this nephrotic syndrome results from an immunotoxic response. Until recently, effects of elemental mercury vapour on the kidney had been reported only at doses higher than those associated with the onset of signs and symptoms from the central nervous system. New studies have, however, reported kidney effects at lower exposure levels. Experimental studies on animals have shown that inorganic mercury may induce auto-immune glomerulonephritis in all species tested, but not in all strains, indicating a genetic predisposition. A consequence of an immunological etiology is that, in the absence of dose-response studies for groups of immunologically sensitive individuals, it is not scientifically possible to set a level for mercury (e.g., in blood or urine) below which (in individual cases) mercury-related symptoms will not occur.

Both metallic mercury vapour and mercury compounds have given rise to contact dermatitis. Mercurial pharmaceuticals have been responsible for Pink disease in children, and mercury vapour exposure may be a cause of "Kawasaki" disease. In some studies, but not in others, effects on the menstrual cycle and/or fetal development have been reported. The standard of published epidemiological studies is such that it remains an open question whether mercury vapour can adversely affect the menstrual cycle or fetal development in the absence of the well-known signs of mercury intoxication.

Recently, there has been an intense debate on the safety of dental amalgams and claims have been made that mercury from amalgam may cause severe health hazards. Reports describing different types of symptoms and signs and the results of the few epidemiological studies produced are inconclusive.

2. IDENTITY, PHYSICAL AND CHEMICAL PROPERTIES, ANALYTICAL METHODS

2.1 Identity

This monograph focuses on the risk to human health from the compounds of inorganic mercury. Other forms of mercury are discussed where they are relevant to the full evaluation of human health risks, e.g., the metabolic transformation of methylmercury to inorganic mercury.

Elemental mercury has the CAS registry number 7439-97-6 and a relative atomic mass of 200.59. There are three states of inorganic mercury: Hg^0 (metallic), Hg_2^{++} (mercurous), and Hg^{++} (mercuric) mercury. The mercurous and mercuric states form numerous inorganic and organic chemical compounds. Organic forms are those in which mercury is attached covalently to at least one carbon atom.

2.2 Physical and chemical properties

In its elemental form, mercury is a heavy silvery liquid at room temperature. At 20 °C the specific gravity of the metal is 13.456 and the vapour pressure is 0.16 Pa (0.0012 mmHg). Thus, a saturated atmosphere at 20 °C contains approximately 15 mg/m³. This concentration is 300 times greater than the recommended health-based occupational exposure limit of 0.05 mg/m³ (WHO, 1980).

Mercurials differ greatly in their solubilities. Solubility values in water are: elemental mercury (30 °C), 2 μg/litre; mercurous chloride (25 °C), 2 mg/litre; mercuric chloride (20 °C), 69 g/litre (Linke, 1958; CRC, 1972). The solubility of methylmercury chloride in water is higher than that of mercurous chloride by about three orders of magnitude, this being related to the very high solubility of the methylmercury cation in water (Linke, 1958; Clarkson et al., 1988b). Certain species of mercury are soluble in non-polar solvents. These include elemental mercury and the halide compounds of alkylmercurials (Clarkson et al., 1988b).

From the biochemical point of view the most important chemical property of mercuric mercury and alkylmercurials is their high affinity for sulfhydryl groups.

Hursh (1985) showed that mercury vapour is more soluble in plasma, whole blood, and haemoglobin than in distilled water or isotonic saline.

The following speciation among mercury compounds has been proposed by Lindqvist et al. (1984), where V indicates volatile species, R water-soluble particle-borne reactive species, and NR non-reactive species:

V: Hg^0 (elemental mercury), $(CH_3)_2Hg$

R: Hg^{2+}, HgX_2, HgX_3^-, and HgX_4^{2-} (where X = OH^-, Cl^-, or Br^-), HgO on aerosol particles, Hg^{2+} complexes with organic acids.

NR: CH_3Hg^+, CH_3HgCl, CH_3HgOH, and other organomercuric compounds, $Hg(CN)_2$, HgS, and Hg^{2+} bound to sulfur in fragments of humic matter.

The main volatile form in air is elemental mercury, but dimethylmercury may also occur (Slemr et al., 1981).

Uncharged complexes, such as $HgCl_2$ and CH_3HgOH, occur in the gaseous phase, but are also relatively stable in fresh water (snow and rain as well as standing or flowing water). $HgCl_4^{2-}$ is the dominant form in sea water.

2.3 Conversion factors

1 ppm = 1 mg/kg = 5 μmol/kg
1 mol creatinine = 113.1 g creatinine

2.4 Analytical methods

Detailed information relating to analytical methods was given in Environmental Health Criteria 1: Mercury (WHO, 1976) and in Environmental Health Criteria 101: Methylmercury (WHO, 1990). This monograph contains further information concerning the sampling and analysis of urine and air, the most frequently studied media for evaluation of exposure to inorganic mercury. A summary of the commonly used analytical methods is given in Table 1. More advanced methods, such as inductively coupled plasma atomic emission spectrometry and spark source mass spectrometry, are described in Kneip & Friberg (1986).

Table 1. Analytical methods for the determination of mercury

Media	Speciation	Analytical method	Detection limit (ng Hg/g)	Comments	References
Food, tissues	total mercury	atomic absorption	2.0	method has many adaptations (see Peter & Strunc, 1984)	Hatch & Ott (1968)
Blood, urine	total mercury inorganic mercury	atomic absorption	0.5	also estimates organic mercury as difference between total and inorganic	Magos (1971); Magos & Clarkson (1972)
Blood, urine hair, tissues	total mercury inorganic mercury	atomic absorption	2.5	automated form of the method of Magos (1971)	Farant et al. (1981)
Blood, urine hair, tissues	total mercury inorganic mercury	atomic absorption	4.0	automated form of the method of Magos (1971)	Coyle & Hartley (1981)
All media	total mercury	neutron activation	0.1	reference method (review)	WHO (1976)

2.4.1 *Analysis, sampling, and storage of urine*

For routine analysis, various forms of flameless atomic absorption spectrophotometry (AAS) are used. The "Magos" selective atomic absorption method determines both total and inorganic mercury and, by difference, organic mercury. The neutron activation procedure is regarded as the most accurate and sensitive procedure and is usually used as the reference method.

Blood samples are best collected in "vacutainers" containing heparin (without mercury compounds as preservative) (WHO, 1980) and stored at 4 °C prior to analysis. This method of collection is especially important if mercury levels in plasma and red blood cells are to be measured. Blood samples can usually be stored for one or two days before haemolysis becomes significant (Clarkson et al., 1988c).

The sampling and storage of urine have been discussed in detail by Clarkson et al. (1988c). It is important to avoid contamination of urine samples; special cleaning procedures and the use of metal-free polyethylene containers have been recommended.

As a rule, urine is saturated with several inorganic salts. Precipitates are sometimes seen in freshly voided samples and are normally present in urine samples that have been stored at low temperature (1-4 °C). To lessen problems of precipitates, urine samples should be homogenized by shaking before analysis. Alternatively, a strong acid, preferably hydrochloric acid, can be added to the urine sample to lower pH and increase the solubility of the salts.

Bacterial growth is rapid in urine at room temperature. Even urine samples from healthy people become overgrown with bacteria after only a few hours. If urine samples are frozen (to below -20 °C), bacterial growth is reduced substantially. Bacteria may reduce some mercury compounds to elemental mercury, which might give rise to significant losses of mercury by volatilization (WHO, 1976). Bactericidal substances, such as sodium azide, may be added to urine samples. However, sodium azide is a strong reducing agent and may form Hg^0 from Hg^{2+}. The addition of 1 g sulfamic acid and 0.5 ml of a detergent (Triton X-100) to 500 ml of urine produces stable urine samples at room temperature for at least one month (Skare, 1972).

Even when the rate of metal excretion is constant, metal concentration in urine varies according to the urine flow rate (Diamond, 1988). It is therefore necessary to adjust the measured concentrations of metals in spot urine samples for variations in the urine flow rate. This can be done by correcting for urine relative density or osmolality or by dividing by the concentration of creatinine in the urine sample. Another alternative is the use of timed urine specimens (e.g., 4 h or 8 h). If the concentration of a substance is standardized to a constant relative density (usually 1.018 or 1.024), the basis of correction chosen profoundly changes the figures obtained. Correction to 1.024 gives values 33% higher than correction to 1.018 (Aitio, 1988). Furthermore, many chemicals, including mercury, exhibit diurnal variation in concentration (Piotrowski et al., 1975). Correction using creatinine values has the advantage that the mercury concentration will be independent of hydration status.

2.4.2 Analysis and sampling of air

Analytical methods for mercury in air may be divided into instant reading methods and methods with separate sampling and analysis stages (WHO, 1976).

One instant reading method is based on the "cold vapour atomic absorption" (CVAA) technique, which measures the absorption of mercury vapour by ultra-violet light using a wave length of 253.7 nm. Most of the AAS procedures have a detection limit in the range of 2 to 5 μg mercury/m^3.

Another instant reading method that has been used increasingly in recent years is a special type of gold amalgamation technique. This method has been used in a number of studies for evaluating the release of elemental mercury vapour in the oral cavity from amalgam fillings (Svare et al., 1981; Vimy & Lorscheider, 1985a,b). McNerney et al. (1972) gave a detailed description of the method, which is based on an increase in the electrical resistance of a thin gold film after adsorption of mercury vapour. The detection limit is 0.05 ng mercury. Within the range of 0.5 to 25 ng, the relative standard deviation was found to vary between 3 and 10% when 15 samples from each of 6 mercury vapour standards were examined. At higher mercury concentrations, the films become saturated with mercury and precision decreases. It is possible to correct for this saturation with a calibration curve. However, there are no data on the accuracy of the method when used in actual field studies, such as the ones by Svare et al. (1981) or Vimy & Lorscheider (1985a,b).

In an analytical method based on separate sampling and analysis, the air is sampled in two bubblers in series, containing sulfuric acid and potassium permanganate (WHO, 1976). The mercury is subsequently determined by CVAA. With this method the *total* mercury in the air is measured, not just mercury vapour. Another sampling technique uses solid absorbants. Different amalgamation techniques using gold have been shown to have good collection efficiency for mercury vapour (McCammon et al., 1980; Dumarey et al., 1985; Skare & Engqvist, 1986). Roels et al. (1987) used a filter with two layers of hopcalite (a mixture of metal oxides that can absorb metals) to collect the mercury. After solubilization, the mercury was analysed by a CVAA technique. It was necessary also to measure blanks of hopcalite and scrubbing solution. Large variations were found for background mercury contamination of hopcalite from batch to batch (6-93 ng mercury per 200 mg hopcalite).

Sampling of air for mercury analysis can be made by static samplers or by personal monitoring. Personal samplers are recommended. A study by Roels et al. (1987) compared results obtained with the use of static samplers with results from personal samplers. In most of the workplaces, personal samplers yielded higher exposure levels (time-weighted averages) than did static samplers (see section 6.5.2).

2.4.3 Quality control and quality assurance

General considerations of quality control and quality assurance have been recommended by WHO (UNEP/WHO, 1984; WHO, 1986; Aitio, 1988). At a recent conference on "Biological Monitoring of Toxic Metals" (Friberg, 1988), a

WHO approach based on a GEMS programme (Vahter, 1982) was described in detail. Specific quality control programmes for mercury in hair using the GEMS approach have been described (Lind et al., 1988). Roels et al. (1987) successfully used another regression method when analysing mercury in urine.

In almost any quality control programme, there is a need for reference materials containing the metal in concentrations covering the expected working range of monitoring samples. Several reference materials are commercially available for both environmental samples and for urine and blood (Muramatsu & Parr, 1985; Parr et al., 1987; Rasberry, 1987; Parr et al., 1988; Okamoto, 1988). The following are suppliers of reference materials: NIST (Office of Standard Reference Materials, National Institute of Standards and Technology, Rm. B311, Chemistry Bldg., Gaithersburg, MD 20899, USA), IAEA (International Atomic Energy Agency, Analytical Quality Control Services, Laboratory Seibersdorf, A-1400 Vienna), BCR (Community Bureau of Reference, Commission of the European Communities, 200 Rue de la Loi, B-1049 Brussels, Belgium); NIES (National Institute for Environmental Studies, Japan Environment Agency, P.O. Yatabe, Tsukuba Ibaraki 300-21, Japan), NRCC (National Research Council Canada, Division of Chemistry, Ottawa, K1A OR6, Canada), Nycomed AS Diagnostics (P.O. Box 4220, Torshov, 0401 Oslo 4, Norway), Behring Institute (P.O. Box 1140, D-3550 Marburg 1, Germany), Kaulson Laboratories Inc. (691 Bloomfield Avenue, Caldwell, New Jersey 07006, USA). However, the available reference materials do not cover the demand for different mercury species, biological media or for different concentrations. Only NRCC has a reference material (fish) for total mercury and for methylmercury.

3. SOURCES OF HUMAN AND ENVIRONMENTAL EXPOSURE

3.1 Natural occurrence

The major natural sources of mercury are the degassing of the earth's crust, emissions from volcanoes, and evaporation from natural bodies of water (National Academy of Sciences, 1978; Nriagu, 1979; Lindqvist et al., 1984). The most recent estimates indicate that natural emissions are of the order of 2700-6000 tonnes per year (Lindberg et al., 1987).

The earth's crust is also an important source of mercury for bodies of natural water. Some of this mercury is undoubtedly of natural origin, but some may have been deposited from the atmosphere and may ultimately have been generated by human activities (Lindqvist et al., 1984). Thus, it is difficult to assess quantitatively the relative contributions of natural and anthropogenic mercury to run-off from land to natural bodies of water. Data concerning mercury in the general environment and in food have been reviewed in Environmental Health Criteria 101: Methylmercury (WHO, 1990).

3.2 Man-made sources

The worldwide mining of mercury is estimated to yield about 10 000 tonnes/year. Mining activities result in losses of mercury through the dumping of mine tailings and direct discharges to the atmosphere. The Almaden mercury mine in Spain, which accounts for 90% of the total output of the European Community, was expected to produce 1380 tonnes in 1987 (Seco, 1987). Other important sources are the combustion of fossil fuel, the smelting of metal sulfide ores, the refining of gold (sometimes under very primitive conditions), the production of cement, refuse incineration, and industrial metal applications. The emissions of mercury to the atmosphere in Sweden in 1984 were estimated to be as follows (in kg/year): incineration of household waste (3300), smelting (900), chloralkali industry (400), crematories (300), mining (200), combustion of coal and peat (200), other sources (200) (Swedish

Environmental Protection Board, 1986). Analogous data for the estimated atmospheric emissions of mercury in the United Kingdom were (in kg/year): fossil fuel combustion (25 500), production and use of articles containing mercury (10 100), municipal waste incineration (5900), non-ferrous metal production (5000), cement manufacture (2500), iron and steel production (1800), sewage sludge incineration (500) (Dean & Suess, 1985). In developing countries the emissions from industry and mining may be much greater. For example, the emission to water from one single chloralkali plant in Nicaragua in 1980 was 24 kg per day (9 tonnes/year) (Velasquez et al., 1980). It was estimated that 450 g of mercury was emitted per tonne of soda produced in six chloroalkali plants in Argentina, and the quantity of mercury released in the environment was about 86 tonnes/year (Gotelli, 1989).

The total global release of mercury to the atmosphere due to human activities has been estimated to be of the order of 2000-3000 tonnes/year (Lindberg et al., 1987; Pacyna, 1987). It should be stressed that there are considerable uncertainties in the estimated fluxes of mercury in the environment and in its speciation. Concentrations in the unpolluted atmosphere and in natural bodies of water are so low that they are near the limit of detection of current analytical methods, even for the determination of total mercury.

Although amounts of mercury resulting from human activities may be quite small relative to global emissions, the anthropogenic release of elemental metal mercury into confined areas was the source of the poisoning outbreaks in Minamata and Niigata (WHO, 1976).

3.3 Uses

A major use of mercury is as a cathode in the electrolysis of sodium chloride solution to produce caustic soda and chlorine gas, which has important uses in the paper-pulp industry. It should be noted that all the electrolytic products (hydrogen, chlorine, sodium hydroxide, sodium hypochlorite, and hydrochloric acid) are contaminated with mercury (Gotelli, 1989). These substances are important in the economy of other industrial activities and the presence of mercury can contaminate other products. About 50 tonnes of liquid metal are used in each manufacturing plant. In most industrialized countries, stringent procedures have been taken to reduce losses of mercury. Mercury is widely used in the electrical industry (lamps, arc rectifiers, and mercury battery cells), in control instruments in the home and industry (switches, thermostats, barometers), and in other laboratory and medical instruments. It is also widely used in the dental profession for tooth amalgam fillings. Other therapeutic agents, such as teething powders, ointments, and laxatives, contain inorganic mercury (ATSDR, 1989), as do some antihistaminic preparations sold in Italy (EDIMED, 1989). Organic mercury compounds continue to be used in antifouling and mildew-proofing latex paints and to control fungus infections of seeds, bulb plants, and vegetation. The World Health Organization has warned against the use of alkylmercury compounds in seed dressing (WHO, 1976).

One of the uses of liquid metallic mercury that may have a serious impact on health is the extraction of gold from ore concentrates or from recycled gold articles. Reports from China (Wu et al., 1989) indicate high exposure in the vicinity of "cottage industry" operations of this type, and Villaluz (1988) reported that 50 000 people may be exposed around small scale gold mining operations in Indonesia, Kampuchea, the Philippines, and Viet Nam. The same problem also occurs in Brazil and Colombia. The release of elemental mercury from these activities is about 120 tonnes/year in Brazil (Gotelli, 1989).

3.4 Dental amalgam in dentistry

WHO (1976) estimated that in industrial countries about 3% of the total consumption of mercury was used for dental amalgam. Amalgam has been used extensively as a tooth-filling material for more than 150 years and accounts for 75-80% of all single tooth restorations (Bauer & First, 1982; Wolff et al., 1983). It has been estimated that each American dentist in private practice uses on average 0.9-1.4 kg of amalgam per year (Naleway et al., 1985).

Most conventional silver amalgams consist of a 1:1 mixture of metallic mercury and an alloy powder consisting of silver (about 70% by weight), tin (about 25%), and smaller amounts of copper (1-6%) and zinc (0-2%). A modern type of silver amalgam is also available, containing higher amounts of copper (up to about 25%). At the time of trituration (mixing), the amalgam generally contains similar weights of alloy powders and mercury. Excess mercury (< 5%) is removed immediately before or at the condensation of the plastic amalgam mix in the prepared tooth cavity. The amalgam begins to set within minutes of insertion and therefore needs to be carved to satisfactory anatomic form within this period of time. Finishing (e.g., polishing) with rotating instruments can take place after setting for 24 h, but continuing hardening of amalgam restorations takes place over many months (ADA, 1985; Enwonwu, 1987; SOS, 1987).

Previously, amalgam was usually prepared with mortar and pestle. The amalgam mixture was thereafter placed on a cloth filter and squeezed to expel excess mercury. This method of handling amalgam easily vapourizes mercury and there is also a risk of spillage. The technique is still in use in some countries (section 9.5.2.2). The modern, safer method for the preparation of amalgam involves mixing the alloy with mercury in a sealed capsule. This decreases the occupational exposure substantially (Harris et al., 1978; Skuba, 1984).

A second type of dental amalgam is the so-called "copper amalgam" used mostly in paediatric dentistry until a few decades ago. This material contained 60-70% mercury and 30-40% copper, and was prepared by open heating in the dental surgery. This process naturally gave rise to considerable occupational mercury vapour exposure. Copper amalgams were easier to retain in dental cavities because of their higher initial plasticity than silver amalgams. Contrary to silver amalgam fillings, copper amalgam undergoes easily detectable dissolution with time. This solubilization was, for some time, actually considered an advantage because of the associated bactericidal effects (SOS, 1987).

A source of mercury loss to the atmosphere is the release of metallic mercury vapour during the cremation of cadavers. Crematories are often located in densely populated areas and do not have high chimneys. All the mercury from amalgam fillings vapourizes during the cremation, as the temperature is above 800 °C. In a Swedish study, it has been estimated that 170-180 kg of metallic mercury is released annually from a total of about 50 000 cremations per year (Mörner & Nilsson, 1986). The use of amalgam in Sweden is estimated to be 5-7.5 tonnes per year (SOS, 1987), compared with 90-100 tonnes in the USA (Wolff et al., 1983; Naleway et al., 1985). It is difficult to esti-mate the global release of mercury vapour from cremation due to uncertainties about dental status at the time of death in relation to frequency of cremations.

3.5 Mercury-containing cream and soap

Mercury-containing cream and soap has for a long time been used by dark-skinned people to obtain a lighter skin tone, probably due to inhibition of pigment formation. There are mainly two types of products distributed for this purpose: skin-lightening creams and skin-lightening soaps. This subject has recently been reviewed by Berlin (personal communication to the IPCS by M. Berlin).

The distribution of the two products is now banned in the European Economic Community, in North America, and in many African states. Mercury-containing soap is, however, manufactured in several European countries and sold as germicidal soap to the Third World, and it has frequently been found in European cities with a substantial black population, such as London and Brussels. This implies that the mercury-containing soap manufactured in Europe has been re-imported illegally from African countries.

English community health authorities (Lambeth, 1988) have identified several brands of soap containing mercury. The soaps have been analysed and contain typically 1-3% of mercuric iodide. There are also skin-lightening creams containing ammoniated mercury from 1-5% (Marzulli & Brown, 1972) or 5-10% (Barr et al., 1973). Both the soap and the cream are applied on the skin, allowed to dry on the skin surface, and left overnight.

4. ENVIRONMENTAL TRANSPORT, DISTRIBUTION, AND TRANSFORMATION

There is a well-recognized global cycle for mercury, whereby emitted mercury vapour is converted to soluble forms (e.g., Hg^{++}) and deposited by rain onto soil and water. Mercury vapour has an atmospheric residence time of between 0.4 and 3 years, whereas soluble forms have residence times of a few weeks. Transport in soil and water is thus limited and deposition within a short distance is highly likely.

The change in mercury speciation from inorganic to methylated forms is the first step in the aquatic bioaccumulation process. Methylation can occur non-enzymatically or through microbial action. Once methylmercury is released, it enters the food chain by rapid diffusion and tight binding to proteins. It attains its highest levels, through food-chain biomagnification, in the tissues of such predatory species as freshwater trout, pike, and bass and marine tuna, swordfish, and shark. The ratio of the methylmercury concentration in fish tissue to the concentration of inorganic mercury in water is usually between 10 000 and 100 000 to one. Levels of selenium in the water may affect the availability of mercury for uptake into aquatic biota. Reports from Sweden and Canada point to the likelihood of increased methylmercury concentration in fish after the construction of artificial water reservoirs (WHO, 1990).

5. ENVIRONMENTAL LEVELS AND HUMAN EXPOSURE

The general population is primarily exposed to mercury from dental amalgam and the diet. However, depending upon the level of contamination, air and water can contribute significantly to the daily intake of total mercury. In most foodstuffs, mercury is usually in the inorganic form and below the limit of detection (20 ng mercury/g fresh weight). The exceptions are fish and fish products, which are the main source of methylmercury in the diet. Levels greater than 1.2 mg/kg are often found in the edible portion of shark, swordfish, and Mediterranean tuna. Similar levels in pike, walleye, and bass taken from polluted fresh water have been identified. Table 2 indicates the average daily intake and retention of total mercury and mercury compounds in the general population not occupationally exposed to mercury.

The level of mercury in fish, even for humans consuming small amounts (10-30 g of fish/day), can markedly affect the intake of methylmercury and, thus, of total mercury. The weekly consumption of 200 g of fish having 500 μg mercury/kg will result in the intake of 100 μg mercury (predominantly methylmercury). This amount is one-half of the tolerable recommended weekly intake (WHO, 1989).

The subject of human mercury dietary exposure has been discussed in previous Environmental Health Criteria monographs (WHO, 1976, 1990). This section emphasizes human exposure to inorganic mercury from dental amalgam and skin-lightening creams and soaps among the general population, and occupational exposure due to the use of amalgam in dentistry. Industrial exposure was described in detail in WHO (1976); more recent information is discussed in section 9.

5.1 General population exposure

5.1.1 Exposure from dental amalgam

5.1.1.1 Human studies

The release of mercury vapour from dental amalgam fillings has been known for a very long time (Stock,

Table 2. Estimated average daily intake and retention (µg/day) of total mercury and mercury compounds in the general population not occupationally exposed to mercury[a]

Exposure	Elemental mercury vapour	Inorganic mercury compounds	Methylmercury
Air	0.030 (0.024)	0.002 (0.001)	0.008 (0.0064)
Food			
Fish	0	0.600 (0.042)	2.4 (2.3)
Non-fish	0	3.6 (0.25)	0
Drinking-water	0	0.050 (0.0035)	0
Dental amalgams	3.8-21 (3-17)	0	0
Total	3.9-21 (3.1-17)	4.3 (0.3)	2.41 (2.31)

[a] From: Environmental Health Criteria 101: Methylmercury (WHO, 1990).
Values given are the estimated average daily intake; the figures in parentheses represent the estimated amount retained in the body of an adult.
Values are quoted to 2 significant figures.

1939). The next major contribution to this field was that of Frykholm (1957). Using a radioactive mercury tracer, he showed that the insertion of amalgam in both humans and dogs resulted in significant concentrations of mercury in urine and faeces. In humans, the concentration of urinary mercury increased during a 5-day period following the insertion of 4-5 small occlusal fillings. A new higher peak occurred a couple of days after removal of these fillings. Faecal elimination showed a similar pattern, appearing on the second day after amalgam insertion. Another maximum appeared 1-2 days after amalgam removal. Frykholm (1957) also measured the concentration of mercury in the oral cavity during amalgam placement in teeth. Recently, concern over amalgam usage has been revived by the publication of a number of experimental studies showing that, among other elements, inorganic mercury is released from amalgam *in vitro* (Brune, 1981; Brune & Evje, 1985). More importantly, mercury vapour released in the mouth *in vivo* leads to an increased uptake of mercury in body tissues (Gay et al., 1979; Svare et al., 1981; Abraham et al., 1984; Ott et al., 1984; Patterson et al., 1985; Vimy & Lorscheider, 1985a,b; Vimy et al., 1986; Langworth et al., 1988; Nylander et al., 1987, 1989; Berglund et al., 1988; Aronsson et al., 1989). Vimy & Lorscheider (1985b) showed that the release rate of mercury vapour increases dramatically when the amalgam is stimulated by continuous chewing, reaching a plateau within 10 min. After the cessation of chewing, it takes approximately 90 min for the mercury release rate to decline to the basal pre-chewing value (Fig. 1). A confirmatory study has recently been published by Aronsson et al. (1989), who also made daily dose estimates.

Critical reviews have been made of published information on mercury release and exposure from amalgam (Enwonwu, 1987; Friberg & Nylander, 1987; Langan et al., 1987; Mackert, 1987; Olsson & Bergman, 1987; Clarkson et al., 1988a). From these reviews it can be concluded that it is difficult to make accurate quantitative estimations of the mercury release from amalgam and the uptake of mercury by the human body. Problems include uncertainty about analytical quality control, differences in sampling methodology, breathing pattern, dilution with inhaled air, and uncertainty about time since previous meals. Due to

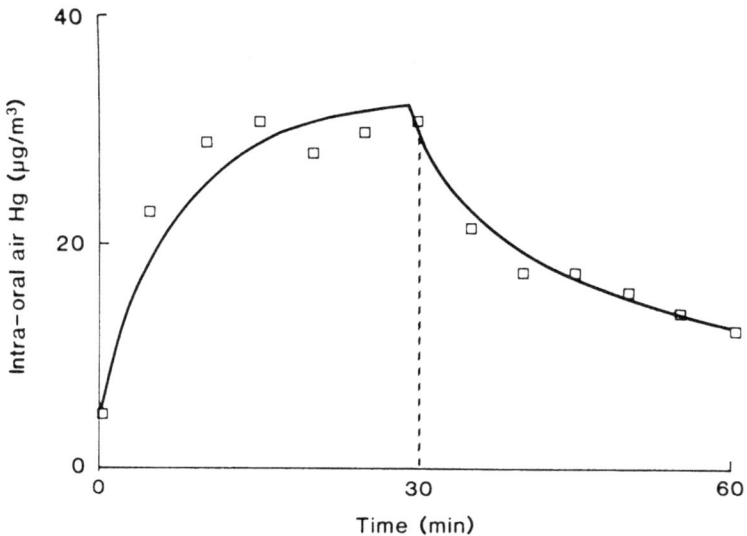

Fig. 1. Mean concentrations of mercury in intra-oral air during 30 min of chewing stimulation, followed by 30 min with no stimulation, in 35 randomly
selected subjects with dental amalgam restorations.
From: Vimy & Lorscheider (1985b).

these factors, some studies may have overestimated and
others underestimated the daily dose of mercury, while
others may have underestimated or overestimated the mercury uptake.

Several studies have correlated the number of dental
amalgam fillings or amalgam surfaces with the mercury
content in brain and kidney tissue from human autopsy.
Subjects with no dental amalgam had a mean mercury level
of 6.7 ng/g (2.4-12.2) in the occipital cortex; whereas,
subjects with amalgams had a mean level of 12.3 ng/g
(4.8-28.7) (Friberg & Nylander, 1987; Nylander et al.,
1987). Amalgam-free subjects had a mean mercury level in
kidneys of 49 ng/g (21-105), whereas subjects with amalgam
fillings had a corresponding level of 433 ng/g (48-810).
In a similar investigation, Eggleston & Nylander (1987)

showed mean mercury levels of 6.7 ng/g (1.9-22.1) and 3.8 ng/g (1.4-7.1) in grey and white brain matter, respectively, in subjects with no amalgam fillings. In subjects with amalgam fillings, mercury levels were 15.2 ng/g (3.0-121.4) and 11.2 ng/g (1.7-110.1) for grey and white matter, respectively. In a more recent extensive study, Schiele (1988) showed a mean brain occipital mercury concentration of 10 ng/g for 44 subjects with an average of 14 amalgam surfaces each. Kidneys from the same subjects showed a sex difference in the mercury concentrations, mean values being 484 ng/g for the 16 females and 263 for the 28 males. Amalgam-free subjects were not included in this study.

Using published experimental data (Svare et al., 1981; Abraham et al., 1984; Patterson et al., 1985; Vimy & Lorsheider, 1985b), the amalgam mercury release rate, average daily mercury uptake, and its steady-state contribution to blood, urine, brain, and kidney were estimated by Clarkson et al. (1988a). These estimations gave brain, kidney, and urine values that are similar to data reported from human studies (brain and kidney autopsy samples: Friberg et al., 1986; Nylander et al., 1987; Schiele, 1988; urine: Nilsson & Nilsson, 1986b; Olstad et al., 1987; Langworth, 1987). A representative illustration of the type of relationship found is given in Fig. 2. Estimates of daily dosages of mercury attributed to amalgam have also been reported by Mackert (1987) and Olsson & Bergman (1987), although they are somewhat lower than those of Clarkson et al. (1988a).

Snapp et al. (1989) studied the blood mercury level before and 18 weeks after the removal of amalgam fillings. After the removal, nine of the ten subjects examined exhibited a statistically significant mean decrease of 1.13 ng ($\pm$ 0.6) mercury/ml in the blood mercury level.

Recently, Molin et al. (1990) studied mercury concentrations in human plasma, erythrocytes, and urine before and up to 12 months after removal of amalgam fillings and replacements with gold alloy restorations. They noted an initial increase in all recorded mercury levels after amalgam removal. About three months thereafter, plasma and erythrocyte levels decreased markedly. A continuous reduction in urine mercury levels took place, reaching a

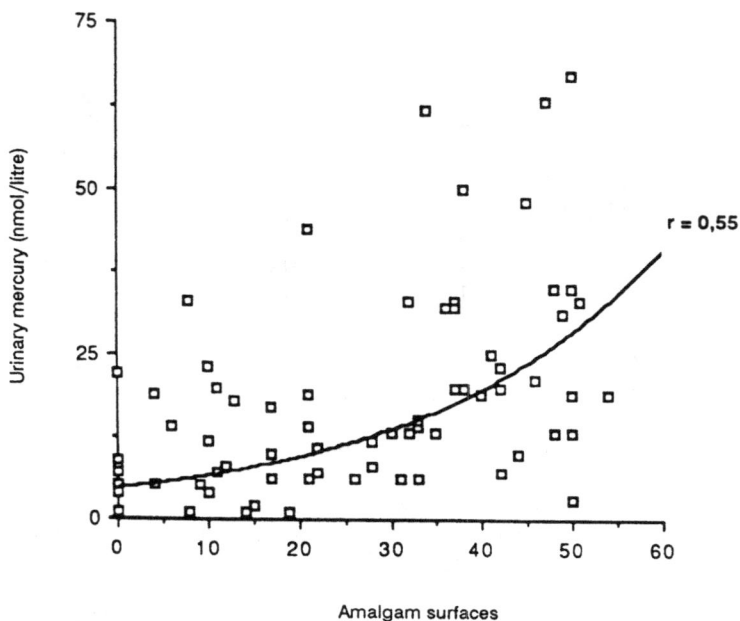

Fig. 2. Relationship between number of amalgam surfaces and urinary mercury concentration. From: Langworth et al. (1988).

plateau of approximately 25% of the pre-removal mercury level within 9 months.

It is important to note that, in the studies cited, both the predicted mercury uptake from amalgam and the observed accumulation of mercury in the body are average values. It is also clear from the original reports that substantial individual variations exist.

5.1.1.2 Animal experiments

Frykholm (1957), using radioactive mercury in amalgam, studied the release and uptake of mercury in dogs and monkeys. He concluded that the mercury exposure from amalgam was essentially limited to the immediate placement procedures. This is in contrast to more recent studies that examined the disposition of radioactive mercury released from amalgam restorations in sheep (Hahn et al., 1989; Vimy et al., 1990a).

Hahn et al. (1989) demonstrated by whole-body image scan that amalgam mercury could be readily visualized in the kidney, liver, jawbone, and gastrointestinal tract after only 29 days of chewing with amalgam. Vimy et al. (1990a) demonstrated that the mercury levels in maternal blood, fetal blood, and amniotic fluid reached a peak within 48 h after amalgam placement and remained at that level for the duration of the studies (140 days). Mercury levels of 4 ng/g in maternal blood and amniotic fluid and of 10 ng/g in fetal blood were found. The erythrocyte/plasma ratios of mercury from amalgam in both the ewe and fetal lamb were less than unity. The maternal urine mercury concentration ranged from 1-10 ng/g during a 16-day period. Approximately 7.7 mg of mercury could be eliminated per day in the faeces.

All tissues examined displayed mercury accumulation. By 29 days, kidney mercury levels rose to approximately 9000 ng/g, and these levels were maintained throughout the duration of the study. A similar pattern was observed in the liver, but the levels remained at approximately 1000 ng/g. The fetal kidney contained mercury levels of 10-14 ng/g, whereas fetal liver had levels of 100-130 ng/g.

The maternal brain (cerebrum, occipital lobe, and thalamus) showed a mercury accumulation ranging from 3-13 ng/g. In the pituitary, thyroid, and adrenal glands, concentrations ranged from approximately 10-100 ng/g. In the fetal cerebrum, occipital cortex, and thalamus the highest levels were approximately 10 ng/g. The fetal pituitary gland had mercury concentrations of more than 100 ng/g, whereas the thyroid and adrenal glands contained less than 10 ng/g.

Milk obtained at lamb parturition or within several days following birth (25-41 days after amalgam placement) contained levels of mercury from dental amalgam that reached as high as 60 ng/g.

Other recent reports indicate that both kidney function (Vimy et al., 1990b) and intestinal bacterial population (Summers et al., 1990) may be affected when animals are exposed to dental amalgam mercury.

5.1.2 Skin-lightening soaps and creams

Elemental mercury and soluble inorganic mercury compounds can penetrate the human skin. Mercury-containing skin-lightening soaps and creams are left on the skin overnight. Therefore, the possibility of substantial mercury exposure exists both via the skin and through inhalation. There are no empirical data showing the relative importance of the different exposure routes, but the evidence indicates that the total exposure to mercury is substantial from these sources. Barr et al. (1973) reported that in a group of 60 African women using skin-lightening creams (5-10% ammoniated mercury), the mean urinary mercury excretion was 109 μg/litre (range: 0-220 μg per litre). A subgroup of 26 women with a nephrotic syndrome had a mean urinary mercury level of 150 μg/litre (range: 90-250 μg/litre). Marzulli & Brown (1972) reported urinary mercury levels from 28 to 600 μg/litre among a group of 6 women who had used skin-lightening cream containing 1-3% ammoniated mercury for two years.

Lauwerys et al. (1987) reported the case of a woman who had recently given birth and who had used during pregnancy and lactation a soap containing 1% mercury as mercuric iodide and a mercury-containing cream. The urinary mercury content of the mother was 784 μg/g creatinine 4 months after the birth at a time when she was still using the soap and cream. Although no mercury-containing cream or soap was used on her baby's skin and the lactation period lasted only one month, the baby's blood (at the age of three months) contained 19 μg/litre and the urine 274 μg/g creatinine.

5.1.3 Mercury in paint

Mercury compounds are added to water-based latex paints to inhibit the growth of bacteria and mould. Several reports have highlighted that mercury vapour can be released from the paint on interior house walls (Hirschman et al., 1963; Jacobs & Goldwater, 1965; Foote, 1972; Sibbett et al., 1972).

A recent study by Agocs et al. (in press) compared homes recently coated with a paint containing a median concentration of 754 mg mercury/litre with homes not coated with a mercury-containing paint to determine whether the recent application of such a paint is associated with elevated concentrations of mercury in air and urine. Air samples from the 19 homes of exposed people contained a median level of 2 $\mu g/m^3$ (range, undetectable to 10 $\mu g/m^3$), while concentrations of mercury in air from 9 homes of unexposed people were below the detection limit of 0.1 $\mu g/m^3$ (p < 0.001). The median urine mercury concentration was higher for the 65 exposed people (8.4 $\mu g/g$ creatinine; range, 2.5-118) than for the 28 unexposed people (1.9 $\mu g/g$ creatinine; range, 0.04-7) (p < 0.001).

5.2 Occupational exposure during manufacture, formulation, and use

Occupational exposure to mercury in chloralkali plants and in mercury mining was reviewed in WHO (1976). In more recent studies, average urine mercury levels of 50-100 μg per litre have been reported (see sections 9.1.2 and 9.2.2).

A NIOSH survey in 1983 of 84 workers in a thermometer factory showed that five workers had urinary mercury levels above 150 $\mu g/g$ creatinine and three workers had levels above 300 $\mu g/g$ creatinine. Personal air sampling showed exposure levels of 26-271 $\mu g/m^3$ (Ehrenberg et al., 1986). Other studies of instrument and thermometer factories in the USA yielded similar results (Price & Wisseman, 1977; Wallingford, 1982; Lee, 1984). In gold and silver refineries in the USA, the mean urinary mercury concentration was 108 $\mu g/litre$ for four regularly exposed workers (Handke & Pryor, 1981).

Recently, particular interest has focused on occupational exposure to mercury in dentistry (see also section 3.2). Several studies made during the period 1960-1980 have reported average levels of mercury vapour in dental clinics ranging between 20 and 30 $\mu g/m^3$ air, and certain clinics have been found to have levels of 150-170 $\mu g/m^3$ (Joselow et al., 1968; Gronka et al., 1970; Buchwald, 1972; Schneider, 1974). Some of these studies also reported the urine mercury levels of dental personnel. Joselow et al. (1968) found an average urinary mercury concentration of 40 µg/litre among 50 dentists, some values exceeding 100 µg/litre. These levels are similar to the urinary mercury concentrations reported by Gronka et al. (1970) and Buchwald (1972).

Kelman (1978) reported statistically significantly higher urine mercury levels among dental assistants (38 µg/litre) than among dentists (22 µg/litre). On the other hand, Nixon et al. (1981) found only small differences between dentists and dental assistants. The average environmental mercury exposure in 200 clinics studied was 11 µg/m³ (with a range from 0 to 82 µg/m³), while the mean urine mercury concentration was 26 µg/litre (2-149 µg/litre).

In a nationwide American study by Naleway et al. (1985), the average mercury level in urine sampled between 1975 and 1983 from 4272 dentists was 14.2 µg/litre (SD ± 25.4 µg/litre; the frequency distribution did not resemble a normal distribution), the range being 0-556 µg per litre. In 4.9% of the samples, levels were above 50 µg/litre, and above 100 µg/litre in 1.3% of samples. The wide range of values was probably due to the sampling techniques, methodological problems, and variations in occupational exposures to amalgam.

In a similar Norwegian study, Jokstad (1987) reported that 2% of a group of 672 dentists had urine mercury levels greater than 20 µg/litre. The highest recorded value in this group was 50 µg/litre.

Recently Nilsson & Nilsson (1986a,b) reported a comparatively low mercury level (4 µg/m³) in the air of private dental clinics. The median urine mercury concentration was 6 µg/litre (range: 1-21 µg/litre) for dentists and 7 µg/litre (range: 1-70 µg/litre) for dental assistants. In a Belgian study of dentists by Huberlant et al. (1983), the mean urine mercury concentration was also relatively low (11.5 µg/g creatinine).

Dentists and dental assistants may be momentarily exposed to high local peaks of mercury vapour during insertion, polishing, and removal of amalgam fillings, especially if adequate protective measures are not taken

(Frykholm, 1957; Buchwald, 1972; Cooley & Barkmeier, 1978; Reinhardt et al., 1983; Richards & Warren, 1985). Richards & Warren (1985) reported mercury vapour concentrations approaching 1000 $\mu g/m^3$ in the breathing zone of dentists not using coolants or adequate aspiration techniques during operative procedures. The corresponding concentrations when proper measures were used were approximatively ten times lower (110 $\mu g/m^3$).

When Battistone et al. (1976) analysed the blood mercury level of 1389 American dentists, the mean value was 9.8 μg/litre (18 dentists having levels above 30 μg per litre). In a study of 380 American dentists, Brady et al. (1980) reported a mean concentration of 8.5 μg per litre, 7.4% of the participants having blood mercury levels greater than 15 μg/litre. These levels were found to decrease within 16 h after termination of exposure. This finding agrees with the documented short biological half-time in blood for the majority of the mercury (see section 6.5).

These studies suffered from variations in the sampling techniques, the analytical techniques, and the occupational exposure of the participants. Although the extent of occupational exposure could be evaluated from mercury concentrations found in critical organs, few data are available in the literature. Kosta et al. (1975) reported levels of mercury in the central nervous system and the kidneys of deceased mercury miners several years after cessation of exposure. Average levels of 700 $\mu g/kg$ wet weight of brain (SD $\pm$ 640 $\mu g/kg$) were, for example, reported in six cases. In the same group plus an additional miner, pituitary mercury levels were reported to be as high as 27 100 $\mu g/kg$ (SD $\pm$ 14 900 $\mu g/kg$). Non-exposed controls showed mean brain levels of 4.2 μg per kg (SD $\pm$ 2.6 $\mu g/kg$, n = 5), mean pituitary levels of 40 μg per kg (SD $\pm$ 26 $\mu g/kg$, n = 6), and mean kidney levels of 140 $\mu g/kg$ (SD $\pm$ 160 $\mu g/kg$, n = 7) (see also sections 9.1.1 and 9.2.1).

A Swedish study of seven former dentists and one dental nurse reported elevated concentrations of mercury in the pituitary gland and occipital lobe cortex (Nylander et al., 1989). Values of up to 4000 $\mu g/kg$ wet weight were observed in the pituitary gland, and of up to

300 μg/kg in the occipital lobe cortex. Two of the subjects were 80 years old and had been retired for several years. High mercury levels were also noted in the kidneys and thyroid. In one subject, the thyroid concentration was 28 000 μg/kg despite several years retirement.

6. KINETICS AND METABOLISM

There are major differences in the kinetics and metabolism of the various mercury species. Metallic mercury is rapidly oxidized to inorganic mercury compounds in the body. However, its kinetics and membrane permeability are different from those of mercuric mercury. Also methylmercury can be converted to inorganic mercury *in vivo* (WHO, 1990). Thus, the ultimate fate of absorbed mercury compounds will depend on their chemical transformation in the body as well as the kinetics. The details of the kinetics and metabolism of methylmercury have been described in WHO (1990).

6.1 Absorption

6.1.1 Absorption by inhalation

Inhalation of mercury vapour is the most important route of uptake for elemental mercury. Approximately 80% of inhaled mercury vapour is retained. The retention occurs almost entirely in the alveoli, where it is almost 100%. The retained amount is the same whether inhalation takes place through the nose or the mouth (WHO, 1976; Hursh et al., 1976).

The uptake of metallic mercury vapour from inspired air into the blood depends on the dissolution of mercury vapour in the blood as it passes through the pulmonary circulation. The dissolved vapour is then very soon oxidized to Hg^{++}, partly in the red blood cells and partly after diffusion into other tissues. This oxidation occurs under the influence of the enzyme catalase. The oxidation, and in consequence the absorption, of mercury vapour in humans can be reduced considerably by alcohol or the herbicide aminotriazole (WHO, 1976; Halbach & Clarkson, 1978; Magos et al., 1978; Hursh et al., 1980).

WHO (1976) concluded that information on pulmonary retention of inorganic mercury compounds was lacking. Deposition should follow the physical laws governing deposition of aerosols in the respiratory system. Particulates with a high probability of deposition in the upper respiratory tract should be cleared quickly. For particulates deposited in the lower respiratory tract, a longer retention period would be expected, the length depending on solubility, among other factors. In experiments on dogs, approximately 45% of a radioactive mercury(II) oxide aerosol, with a median droplet diameter of 0.16 (± 0.06) μm, was cleared in less than 24 h and the remainder with a half-time of 33 days (Morrow et al., 1964). Radioactivity was detected in blood as well as in urine. The concentration in blood followed the curve of its disappearance from the lungs. The *in vivo* solubility of the particles was found to be of great importance for the clearance during the slow phase. Recent evidence has shown that lung macrophages are able to increase the solubility of only slightly soluble metals (Lundborg et al., 1984; Marafante et al., 1987) and that this is due to a low pH in the phagolysosomes (Nilsen et al., 1988).

Although there are still no data to allow a quantitative evaluation of the absorption of different inorganic mercury compounds, significant absorption must take place directly from the lung and, probably, to some extent from the gastrointestinal tract after mucociliary clearance of non-absorbed mercury.

6.1.2 Absorption by ingestion

Liquid metallic mercury is poorly absorbed. Some data indicate an absorption of less than 0.01% in rats. However, humans who accidently ingested several grams of metallic mercury showed increased blood levels of mercury (WHO, 1976). Metallic mercury has been incorporated into tissues after accidental breakage of intestinal tubes, containers, and thermometers. This has sometimes caused local tissue reactions with or without signs of systemic poisoning (Geller, 1976). The reason for the different types of reactions is not known.

The absorption in humans of inorganic mercuric mercury compounds from foods was estimated by WHO (1976) to be about 7% on average and by Elinder et al. (1988) to be less than 10% (probably about 5%). The data were mainly obtained from tracer studies on human volunteers (Rahola et al., 1973), who received single oral doses of protein-bound inorganic mercuric mercury. Although individual variation was considerable, the proportion of the dose excreted in the faeces during the first 4-5 days was 75-92%.

Absorption in young children may be considerably greater. Kostial et al. (1978, 1983) observed an average absorption in newborn rats of 38% six days after an oral dose of mercuric chloride. The absorption in older animals was only about 1%. As breast milk may contain significant amounts of inorganic as well as organic mercury, this route of exposure should not be overlooked (section 6.4). The low solubility of mercurous chloride limits absorption. However, after prolonged intake the accumulation of mercury in tissues, urinary mercury excretion, and adverse effects indicate that some absorption takes place.

6.1.3 Absorption through skin

Little information was available on skin absorption when WHO (1976) was published, although some animal experiments revealed a certain degree of skin penetration (a few per cent of an aqueous solution of mercuric salts during the first hours of skin application) (Friberg et al., 1961; Skog & Wahlberg, 1964; Wahlberg, 1965). Recent studies on human volunteers (Hursh et al., 1989) indicate that uptake via the skin of metallic mercury vapour is only about 1% of uptake by inhalation. However, it is obvious that the use of skin-lightening creams containing inorganic mercury salts causes substantial absorption and accumulation into the body (section 5.1.2), although there is no information on how much of the mercury is absorbed through the skin and how much is absorbed via other routes.

6.1.4 Absorption by axonal transport

Arvidson (1987) reported an accumulation of mercury from a tracer dose of $^{203}HgCl_2$ in the hypoglossal nuclei of the brain stem of rats after a single injection into the tongue. A similar accumulation was not seen in controls after a similar injection into the gluteus maximus muscle. The author concluded that the results provided evidence of retrograde axonal transport of mercury in the hypoglossal nerve.

6.2 Distribution

From studies on animals and humans (WHO, 1976; Khayat & Dencker, 1983a, 1984; see also sections 8 and 9), it is known that mercury has an affinity for ectodermal and endodermal epithelial cells and glands. It accumulates in, for instance, the thyroid, pituitary, brain, kidney, liver, pancreas, testes, ovaries, and prostate. Within the organs the distribution is not uniform. This explains why biological half-times may differ not only between organs but also within an organ. The kidney is the chief depository of mercury after the administration of elemental mercury vapour or inorganic salts. Based on animal data, 50-90% of the body burden is found in the kidneys. Significant amounts were transported to the brain after exposure of mice and monkeys to elemental mercury vapour. The brain mercury levels were ten times higher than after equal doses of mercuric mercury given intravenously (Berlin & Johansson, 1964; Berlin et al., 1969; WHO, 1976). In rats given daily subcutaneous doses of mercuric chloride for six weeks, only 0.01% of the total dose of mercury was found in the brain, while about 3% of the dose was retained in the kidneys (Friberg, 1956).

The red cell to plasma ratio in humans was approximately 1.0 after exposure to Hg^0 vapour, but was 0.4 after exposure to inorganic mercury salts (WHO, 1976). The ratio may vary, however. Suzuki et al. (1976) observed a red cell to plasma ratio of about 1.5-2 for workers exposed only to mercury vapour, while the corresponding ratio for 6 chloralkali workers (where the exposure may have been to both vapour and inorganic salts) averaged only 0.02. The reason for this extremely low ratio is unknown. In a report by Cherian et al. (1978), a ratio of about 2 was observed during the first few days after exposure of volunteers to metallic mercury vapour.

Jugo (1976) compared the retention of mercuric chloride after a single injection in adult and 2-week-old suckling rats. The whole-body retention 6 days after treatment was significantly higher in the suckling animals, and the accumulation of mercury was 13- and 19-fold higher in the brain and liver, respectively, compared to adult rats. On the other hand, the mercury concentrations in the kidneys were markedly higher in the adult group.

In two pregnant women who had been accidentally exposed to metallic mercury vapour, the concentration of mercury in the infant blood was similar to that in the maternal blood at the time of delivery (Clarkson & Kilpper, 1978). There are no other data on the transfer of inhaled mercury vapour to the fetus in humans.

Based on studies in rodents, elemental mercury vapour easily penetrates the placental barrier and, after oxidation, accumulates in the fetal tissue. Only a fraction of divalent mercury enters the fetus, but it can accumulate in the placenta. Clarkson et al. (1972) found that mercury levels in the fetuses of rats exposed to mercury vapour were 10-40 times higher than in animals exposed to equivalent doses of mercuric chloride. Differences in the penetration of the placental barrier have been confirmed in mice by Khayat & Dencker (1982), who found a 4-fold higher fetal mercury concentration after exposure to metallic mercury vapour than after exposure to mercuric chloride. The uptake of mercury vapour increased with gestational age. Only traces of radioactive mercury were found in embryos at 8 and 10 days of gestation. A distinct accumulation of mercury was seen in the fetal tissue from day 12 of gestation with a pronounced uptake in the fetal liver and heart. The mercury concentration in the CNS was rather low in early and mid gestation but increased just prior to birth (Ogata & Meguro, 1986).

Yoshida et al. (1986, 1987) studied the uptake and distribution of mercury in the fetus of guinea-pigs during late gestation after repeated exposure to 200-300 μg mercury vapour/m^3 2 h/day and after a single exposure for 150 min to 8-11 mg/m^3. Mercury concentrations in fetal brain, lungs, heart, kidneys, and blood were much lower than those in maternal tissues, the concentrations differing by a factor of about 5 in the brain and a factor of up to 100 in the kidneys. Mercury concentrations in fetal liver were up to two times higher than those found in maternal liver. In the fetal liver, more than 50% of the mercury was bound to a metallothionein-like protein with a relative molecular mass of about 10 000 to 12 000. The bulk of the eluted mercury in the maternal liver was associated with a protein of high relative molecular mass. The authors suggested that the fetal metallothionein-like protein plays a role in preventing further distribution of mercury from the liver after *in utero* exposure to mercury vapour.

Mercury distribution in the neonate differs from that in the fetus (Yoshida et al., 1989). A significantly increased level was found in kidney, lung, and brain in neonate guinea-pigs, compared with fetuses, and there was a progressive decrease in liver concentration, with diminishing hepatic metallothionein levels, in the neonates. These results suggest a redistribution of mercury to other tissues in the neonate.

The oxidation of elemental mercury vapour in the body (section 6.1.1) can be reduced considerably (to about 50% of normal values) by moderate amounts of alcohol. In an *in vivo* study, the uptake of labelled mercury into human red cells was reduced by almost a factor of ten by ethanol, while there was an increase in liver mercury concentrations (Hursh et al., 1980). Observations on rats, mice, and monkeys confirm these results (Khayat & Dencker, 1983a,b, 1984). They also show a marked decrease in mercury concentrations in several organs, including the brain. However, somewhat higher concentrations of mercury were observed in the brain and liver of pregnant mice with a congenital catalase deficiency that were exposed for 1 h to metallic mercury vapour during day 18 of gestation (Ogata & Meguro, 1986). The blood mercury concentration in the catalase-deficient mice was only about half of that in the control mice. The uptake in the fetus was 2% of the dose compared to 1.2% for the controls.

Lower mercury levels have been observed in the brain tissue of humans classified as chronic alcohol abusers than in controls (Fig. 3).

6.3 Metabolic transformation

Several forms of metabolic transformation occur:

* oxidation of metallic mercury vapour to divalent mercury;
* reduction of divalent mercury to metallic mercury;
* methylation of inorganic mercury;
* conversion of methylmercury to divalent inorganic mercury.

The oxidation of metallic mercury vapour to divalent ionic mercury (section 6.1.1) takes place very soon after

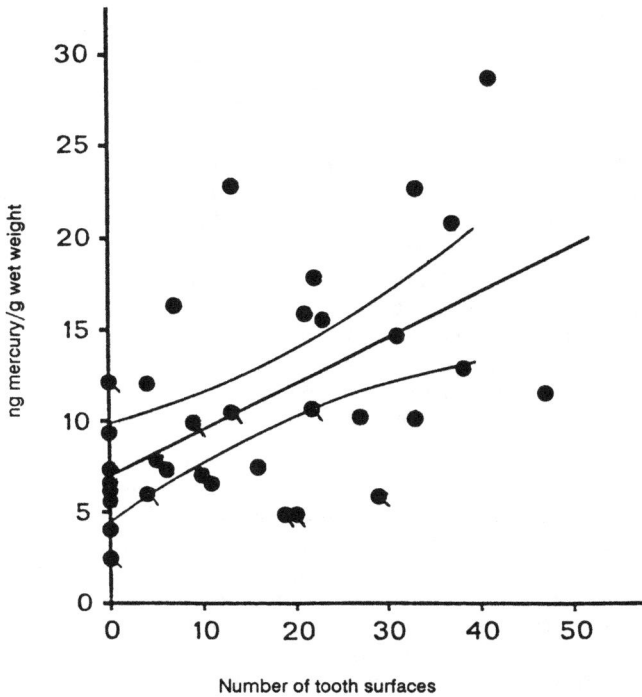

Fig. 3. Number of tooth surfaces containing amalgam in relation to total mercury concentrations in occipital lobe cortex (neutron activation analyses). From: Nylander et al. (1987).
● = Alcoholics; ● = Non-alcoholics.

absorption, but some elemental mercury remains dissolved in the blood long enough (a few minutes) for it to be carried to the blood-brain barrier and the placenta (WHO, 1976). Recent *in vitro* studies on the oxidation of mercury by the blood (Hursh et al., 1988) indicate that because of the short transit time from the lung to the brain almost all the mercury vapour (97%) arrives at the brain unoxidized. Its lipid solubility and high diffusibility allow rapid transit across these barriers. Oxidation of the mercury vapour in brain and fetal tissues converts it to the ionic form, which is much less likely to cross the blood-brain and placental barriers. Thus, oxidation in these tissues serves as a trap to hold the mercury and leads to accumulation in brain and fetal tissues (WHO, 1976).

The reduction of divalent mercury to Hg^0 has been demonstrated both in animals (mice and rats) and humans (WHO, 1976; Dunn et al., 1978, 1981a,b; Sugata & Clarkson, 1979). A small amount of exhaled mercury vapour is the result of this reduction. It is increased in catalase-deficient mice (Ogata et al., 1987) and by alcohol (both *in vitro* and *in vivo*) in both mice and humans (Dunn et. al., 1981a,b). The increased exhalation of mercury vapour in the latter case may be explained by assuming that the oxidation by catalase is less than normal.

It was stated in WHO (1976) that there is no evidence in the literature for the synthesis of organomercury compounds in human or mammalian tissues. Minor methylation may occur *in vitro* by intestinal or oral bacteria (Rowland et al., 1975; Heintze et al., 1983). A slight increase in the concentration of methylmercury in blood and/or urine has been reported among dentists and workers in the chloralkali industry (Cross et al., 1978; Pan et al., 1980; Aitio et al., 1983). These data cannot be taken as evidence of methylation, however, due to lack of analytical quality control and possible confounding by exposure to methylmercury. Chang et al. (1987) did not observe any methylation in a study of dentists.

The conversion of methylmercury to inorganic mercury is considered a key step in the process of excretion of mercury after exposure to methylmercury (WHO, 1990). If the intact molecule of an organomercurial in an organ is more rapidly excreted than inorganic mercury, biotransformation will decrease the overall excretion rate, and the ratio of inorganic to organic mercury in that particular organ will increase with time. The fraction of total mercury present as Hg^{++} will depend on the duration of exposure to methylmercury and/or the time elapsed since cessation of exposure. Even if the demethylation rate is very slow, this process may in the long run give rise to considerable accumulation of inorganic mercury. The ratio of methylmercury to inorganic mercury depends on the rate of demethylation and the clearance half-times of methyl-mercury and inorganic mercury.

After short-term exposure of experimental animals to methylmercury the kidneys usually contain the highest fraction of Hg^{++} in relation to total mercury, while the relative concentration in the brain is low (WHO, 1976). In studies on squirrel monkeys (Berlin et al., 1975), the short-term biotransformation to inorganic mercury was as follows: of the total mercury, about 20% was inorganic in the liver; 50% in the kidney; 30%-85% in the bile; and less than 5% in the brain.

More recent data from long-term studies on monkeys show a different pattern. Mottet & Burbacher (1988) sum-marized a long series of studies on the metabolism and toxicity of methylmercury in monkeys *(Macaca fascicularis)*. The monkeys had been orally exposed to high levels of methylmercury for a period of years and sacrificed during the ongoing exposure. At the end of the exposure period, 10-33% of the mercury in the brain was present in the inorganic form (Lind et al., 1988). In monkeys that had been without mercury exposure for 6 months to almost two years after the same treatment, the relative concentration of inorganic mercury was much higher, i.e. about 90%. Exact half-times for the different compounds could not be established in the absence of data on the concentrations of inorganic and organic mercury in the brain at different time intervals during the accumulation and clearance phases. Recent data by Rice (1989) also demonstrate demethylation in the brain. Female monkeys *(Macaca fascicularis)* were dosed for at least 1.7 years with mercury as methylmercury chloride (10-50 µg/kg per day). After dosing ceased, the blood mercury half-time was about 14 days. Approximately 230 days after cessation of dosing, the monkeys were sacrificed and brain total mercury levels determined. These levels were considered to be at least three orders of magnitude higher than those predicted by assuming the half-time in brain to be the same as that in blood. The author considered the most likely explanation to be demethylation of methylmercury and subsequent binding of inorganic mercury to tissue.

Similar results were recently reported by Hansen et al. (1989) who fed fish contaminated with methylmercury to one Alsatian dog for 7 years. The dog was examined after its death at the age of 12 years, 4 years after the exposure to methylmercury had ceased. Two dogs of the same age and breed served as controls. In the CNS, the mercury was fairly uniformly distributed and 93% was in the inorganic state, whereas the skeletal muscles contained approximately 30% inorganic mercury. The authors concluded that the results demonstrated time-dependent demethylation and suggested a variation in the rate from one type of tissue to another. High levels of mercury were demonstrated by a histochemical method in the liver, thyroid gland, and kidney, whereas practically no mercury was found in any of the organs examined in the control dogs. The distribution of inorganic mercury was determined by a histochemical method for locating mercury in tissue sections. Total mercury was analysed by flameless atomic absorption and organic mercury by GC.

A considerable fraction of the mercury in human brains is reported to be in the form of inorganic mercury. Kitamura et al. (1976) analysed autopsy material from 20 Japanese subjects for total mercury using flameless atomic absorption and for methylmercury using GC. The median concentration of total mercury in the cerebrum was 0.097 mg/kg wet weight and of methylmercury 0.012 mg/kg wet weight. The values for the cerebellum were similar. No analytical quality control data were reported.

In a Swedish autopsy study covering six cases (Friberg et al., 1986; Nylander et al., 1987), about 80% of the mercury in the occipital lobe cortex was inorganic. The concentration of inorganic mercury varied between 3 and 22 μg/kg wet weight. Both total mercury and inorganic mercury were determined by the method of Magos (Magos, 1971; Magos & Clarkson, 1972). For quality control purposes total mercury was also analysed by neutron activation analysis. In this study, however, the concentrations of mercury in the brain were considerably lower than in the Japanese study. As has been discussed in section 5.1.1, an association between the number of amalgam fillings and total mercury concentration in the occipital lobe has been found. Exposure to inorganic mercury from dental fillings could explain the high proportion of inorganic mercury in the Swedish study but not in the Japanese study, as it seems reasonable to assume that the mercury exposure from amalgam should be approximately the same in the two countries. The exposure to methylmercury could, however, easily differ considerably.

Takizawa (1986) reported the total mercury and methylmercury brain concentrations in about 30 humans who had died from 20 days to 18 years after the onset of symptoms of methylmercury poisoning. The total mercury content was measured by flameless atomic absorption spectrophotometry, while methylmercury was analysed by electron capture GLC (Minagawa et al., 1979; Takizawa, 1986). The total mercury content in "acute" cases (autopsy < 100 days after onset of symptoms) was 8.8-21.4 mg/kg and the concentration of methylmercury was 1.85-8.42 mg mercury/kg. The concentrations for the "chronic" cases were 0.35-5.29 mg/kg for total mercury and 0.31-1.02 mg mercury/g for methylmercury. On average, only 28% of the mercury was present as methylmercury in the acute cases and 17% in the chronic cases. Takizawa (1986) also presented data for residents near Minamata Bay and for a non-polluted area. The best estimate from these data is that only 16% and 12%, respectively, of the total mercury was present as methylmercury. Unfortunately, in these reports quality control data were not presented. The authors measured total mercury and methylmercury and assumed that the difference between these analyses was due to inorganic mercury. It could in principle, in whole or in part, also have been methylmercury that was not extracted in the gas chromatographic procedure. Ideally, analyses should be carried out using, for instance, the method by Magos (1971), which measures total mercury and inorganic mercury.

The tissues in the studies by Takizawa (1986) were stored for long periods after fixation with a 10% neutral formalin solution. Miyama & Suzuki (1971) found that the ratio of inorganic to total mercury in the cerebral cortex increased from about 35% (tissues stored frozen) to about 50% after storage in 10% formalin for one year. However, there was no loss of inorganic mercury. Eto et al. (1988) compared results from a small number of analyses of formalin-fixed tissues with results from analyses of frozen tissues. There was no systematic loss related to storage in formaldehyde.

The concentrations of inorganic mercury in the brain, reported in overt cases of methylmercury poisoning, are very high, similar to those observed after toxic exposure to metallic mercury vapour. Whether or not an accumulation of inorganic mercury actually contributed to the toxic effects is not known, but seems unlikely. Even assuming no analytical problems, it should be borne in mind that the methylmercury poisoning usually occurred after relatively short exposure to methylmercury when no significant biotransformation should yet have taken place. However, a comparison of the toxicology of methylmercury with that of ethylmercury, which decomposes significantly more quickly, indicated that cerebellar damage could not be related to inorganic mercury. The higher concentration of inorganic mercury in the brain of ethylmercury-treated rats, compared with methylmercury-treated rats, was associated with less cerebellar damage (Magos et al., 1985). It is more difficult to evaluate the possible long-term effects of inorganic mercury, which slowly accumulates in the brain.

The distribution of ionic mercury in the brain will depend on whether Hg^{++} enters the brain in the ionic form or as a result of *in situ* biotransformation following penetration of the brain barrier by elemental mercury or methylmercury. The toxicological aspects of such possible differences in distribution are not known.

6.4 Elimination and excretion

A small portion of absorbed inorganic mercury is exhaled as metallic mercury vapour, formed by the reduction of Hg^{++} in the tissues (Dunn et al., 1978), but urine and faeces are the principal routes of elimination (WHO, 1976). The urinary route dominates when exposure is high. After exposure to metallic mercury vapour, a small fraction of the mercury in the urine may be present as elemental mercury (Stopford et al., 1978; Yoshida & Yamamura, 1982). One form of depletion is the transfer of maternal mercury to the fetal unit. Thus, inorganic mercury was detected in the amniotic fluid in all but two out of 57 Japanese pregnant women, while organic mercury was found in only 30 women (Suzuki et al., 1977). In a study by Skerfving (1988), it was reported that the concentrations of total mercury in breast milk and in the blood plasma of breast-fed infants were similar to those in the maternal plasma of Swedish fishermen's wives. Although the women were exposed to methylmercury, 80% of mercury excreted in breast milk was in the inorganic form. No formal analytical quality control procedures were applied in the studies where mercury was speciated.

6.5 Retention and turnover

6.5.1 Biological half-time

Only very limited data were available on the biological half-time of inorganic mercury when WHO (1976) was published. Studies on a small number of volunteers had shown that the elimination of mercury, after a single exposure to metallic mercury vapour, followed a single exponential process with an average half-time of 58 days during the first few months after the exposure. Similar data were available from studies involving oral exposure to mercuric mercury. It was pointed out that there had been a few reports of high brain mercury concentrations in workers several years after cessation of exposure to mercury vapour. This indicated that the half-time in brain is longer than that in other organs, although no quantitative estimations were made.

As a result of tracer studies on human volunteers (Nakaaki et al., 1975, 1978; Cherian et al., 1978; Newton & Fry, 1978; Hursh et al., 1980) and animals (Berlin et al., 1975), more data are now available on the kinetics during the first few months after exposure. The elimination of inorganic mercury follows a complicated pattern with biological half-times that differ according to the tissue and the time after exposure. The best estimate is that after short-term exposure to mercury vapour, the first phase of elimination from blood has a half-time of approximately 2-4 days and accounts for about 90% of the mercury. This is followed by a second phase with a half-time of 15-30 days.

In tracer studies on nine human volunteers (Hursh et al., 1976, 1980; Clarkson et al., 1988a) the half-time for most of the mercury in the brain was 19 (± 1.7) days during the first 35 to 45 days. Newton & Fry (1978) found half-times of 23 and 26 days in the head of two subjects accidentally exposed to radioactive mercuric oxide. In a study by Berlin et al. (1975), a steady state was not reached in the brains of squirrel monkeys exposed for two months to mercury vapour. In one study on monkeys *(Macaca fascicularis)* (section 6.3) lasting several years where inorganic mercury accumulated in the brain (probably as a result of demethylation of methylmercury), there was still considerable inorganic mercury in the brain 1-2 years after cessation of exposure (Lind et al., 1988). These results indicate a very long half-time for a fraction of the inorganic mercury in the brain. This is in accordance with data from deceased miners and dentists (section 5.2).

The half-time in the kidneys for inorganic mercury in the studies by Hursh et al. (1976, 1980) was 64 days, about the same as that for the body as a whole. As in the case of the brain, a fraction of the mercury probably has a long biological half-time (section 5.2).

A few attempts to perform a quantitative evaluation of the half-time for inorganic mercury have been made using multicompartment models (Sugita, 1978; Bernard & Purdue, 1984). According to the recommendation of ICRP (1980), the four-compartment model of Bernard & Purdue (1984) included one compartment with a half-time of 27 years. As the basic assumptions are uncertain, the models are uncertain, but may be of value for a possible "worst case" estimation of the retention of inorganic mercury in the brain. The model of Bernard & Purdue (1984) has been used by Vimy et al. (1986) for calculating mercury accumulation in the brain from amalgam fillings (section 5.1). The form of mercury that is responsible for the long biological half-time may be biochemically inactive mercury selenide.

6.5.2 Reference or normal values in indicator media

A considerable amount of information is given in Environmental Health Criteria 101: Methylmercury (WHO, 1990). The mean concentration of total mercury in whole blood (in the absence of consumption of fish with high concentrations of methylmercury) is probably of the order of 5-10 μg/litre, and in hair about 1-2 mg/kg. The average mercury concentration in urine is about 4 μg per litre and in the placenta about 10 mg/kg wet weight, although the individual variation is substantial. One source of the variation in urine levels seems to be exposure from dental amalgam (Fig. 4), while for blood and hair levels fish consumption is the major source of exposure. Increased hair levels may also be due to external contamination.

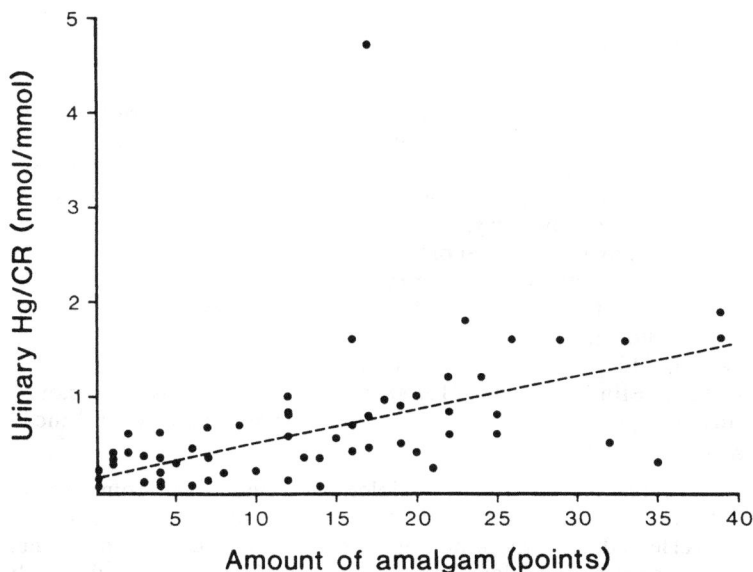

Fig. 4. Creatinine-adjusted urinary mercury values (Hg/CR) in relation to amount of amalgam restoration (amalgam points). Broken line: linear regression line ($r = 0.55$).

There are at present no suitable indicator media that will reflect concentrations of inorganic mercury in the critical organs, the brain or kidney, under different exposure situations. This is to be expected in view of the complicated pattern of metabolism for different mercury compounds. One important consequence is that concentrations of mercury in urine or blood may be low quite soon after exposure has ceased, despite the fact that concentrations in the critical organs may still be high.

There is some information, obtained from subjects not occupationally exposed and with only a moderate fish consumption, on the relationship between exposure to metallic mercury vapour and concentrations of mercury in urine and brain tissue. This relationship (section 5.1) indicates that ongoing long-term exposure to elemental mercury vapour, leading to a mercury absorption of 5-10 μg/day, will result in a mercury excretion in urine of about 5 μg/litre and average mercury concentrations in the occipital lobe cortex and kidney of approximately 10 μg/kg and 500 μg/kg, respectively.

The distribution between blood and hair is well known for different exposure levels of methylmercury, which forms the basis for the use of hair as an indicator media for this compound. There is no corresponding information for inorganic mercury. When high levels of total mercury in hair have been reported, for instance, among dentists exposed to metallic mercury vapour (see e.g. Sinclair et al., 1980; Pritchard et al., 1982; Sikorski et al., 1987), it was not known how much was due to external contamination. In a report on biological monitoring of toxic metals, Elinder et al. (1988) concluded that hair is not a suitable indicator medium for monitoring exposure to inorganic mercury.

There is good epidemiological evidence from occupational exposure that, on a group basis, recent exposure is reflected in the mercury levels in blood and urine. When exposure is low (e.g., from amalgam), it is difficult to find an association between exposure levels and blood concentrations due to confounding exposures to methylmercury in fish. A way to overcome the problem may be to analyse mercury in plasma or speciate the analysis for inorganic mercury (Elinder et al., 1988). The problem of confounding exposures is not so important when analysing urine, as only a very small fraction of absorbed methylmercury is excreted in urine.

Data amassed by Smith et al. (1970) from the chlorine industry were used by WHO (1976) to evaluate the relationship between concentrations of metallic mercury vapour in air and concentrations of mercury in blood and urine. Long-term time-weighted occupational exposure to an average air mercury concentration of 50 μg/m^3 was considered to be associated, on a group basis, with blood mercury levels of approximately 35 μg/litre, and with urinary concentrations of 150 μg/litre. The ratio of urine to air concentrations was re-evaluated by WHO (1980) to be closer to 2.0-2.5 instead of 3.0. The mercury concentrations in air were measured with static samplers. Results from a number of more recent studies have been reported where both static samplers and personal samplers have been used (Ishihara et al., 1977; Lindstedt et al., 1979; Müller et al., 1980; Mattiussi et al., 1982; Roels et al., 1987). Where personal samplers have been used, the ratio between urinary mercury (μg/litre or per g creatinine) and mercury in air (μg/m^3) has as a rule been 1-2. When blood values were reported they were either similar to those given in WHO (1976) or somewhat lower.

In the study by Roels et al. (1987), personal monitoring was used, detailed quality control procedures were implemented and reported, and the examined subjects had been exposed to defined concentrations for at least one year. A good relationship could be established between the daily time-weighted exposure to mercury vapour and the daily level of mercury in blood and urine (Fig. 5). Urinary levels of about 50 μg/g creatinine were seen after occupational exposure to about 40 μg/m^3 of air. Such an exposure would correspond to about 17 μg/litre of blood.

Several studies have reported a correlation between mercury in blood and urine. The results vary considerably and it is not known whether the ratio between concentrations in urine and blood is constant at different exposure levels. At low exposure levels the possibilities of a significant confounding effect on blood levels should always be borne in mind.

On the basis of studies by Smith et al. (1970) and Lindstedt et al. (1979), Skerfving & Berlin (1985) suggested that a urine mercury level of 50 μg/g creatinine is associated with a blood mercury level of 20 μg per litre. Roels et al. (1987) reported a regression equation, where a urine mercury level of 50 μg/g creatinine leads to a blood mercury level of 16 μg/litre.

(a)

n = 34
r = 0.81
p < 0.001
y = 10.2 + 1.01x

(b)

n = 40
r = 0.86
p < 0.001
y = -0.14 + 0.048x

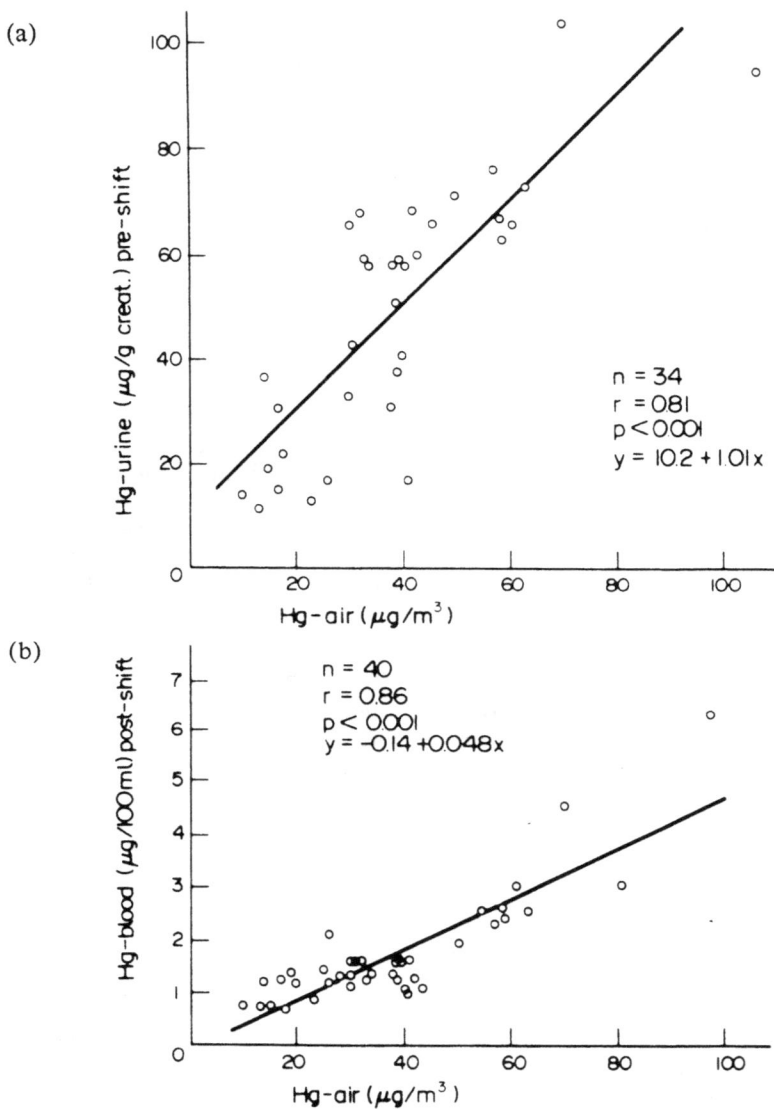

Fig. 5. Relationships between individual daily levels of mercury in air on hopcalite filters by personal sampler and:
(a) those in blood samples taken at the end of the work shift (14.00 h);
(b) those in urine samples collected the following morning (9.00 h). From: Roels et al. (1987).

7. EFFECTS ON ORGANISMS IN THE ENVIRONMENT

This chapter is extracted from the summary of Environmental Health Criteria 86: Mercury - Environmental Aspects (WHO, 1989).

7.1 Uptake, elimination, and accumulation in organisms

Mercuric salts, and, to a much greater extent, organic mercury, are readily taken up by organisms in water. Aquatic invertebrates, and most particularly aquatic insects, accumulate mercury to high concentrations. Fish also take up the metal and retain it in tissues, principally as methylmercury, although most of the environmental mercury to which they are exposed is inorganic. The source of the methylation is uncertain, but there is strong indication that bacterial action leads to methylation in aquatic systems. Environmental levels of methylmercury depend upon the balance between bacterial methylation and demethylation. The indications are that methylmercury in fish arises from this bacterial methylation of inorganic mercury, either in the environment or in bacteria associated with fish gills, surface, or gut. There is little indication that fish themselves either methylate or demethylate mercury. Elimination of methylmercury is slow from fish (with half times in the order of months or years) and from other aquatic organisms. Loss of inorganic mercury is more rapid and so most of the mercury in fish is retained in the form of methylmercury. Terrestrial organisms are also contaminated by mercury, with birds being the best studied. Sea birds and those feeding in estuaries are most contaminated. The form of retained mercury in birds is more variable and depends on species, organ, and geographical site.

7.2 Toxicity to microorganisms

The metal is toxic to microorganisms. Inorganic mercury has been reported to have effects at concentrations of the metal in the culture medium of 5 μg/litre, and organomercury compounds at concentrations at least 10 times lower than this. Organomercury compounds have been used as fungicides. One factor affecting the toxicity of the organometal is the rate of uptake of the metal by cells. Mercury is bound to the cell walls or cell membranes of microorganisms, apparently to a limited number of binding sites. This means that effects are related to cell density as well as to the concentration of mercury in the substrate. These effects are often irreversible, and mercury at low concentrations represents a major hazard to microorganisms.

7.3 Toxicity to aquatic organisms

The organic forms of mercury are generally more toxic to aquatic organisms than the inorganic forms. Aquatic plants are affected by mercury in the water at concentrations approaching 1 mg/litre for inorganic mercury but at much lower concentrations of organic mercury. Aquatic invertebrates vary greatly in their susceptibility to mercury. Generally, larval stages are more sensitive than adults. The 96-h LC_{50}s vary between 33 and 400 μg per litre for freshwater fish and are higher for sea-water fish. However, organic mercury compounds are more toxic. Toxicity is affected by temperature, salinity, dissolved oxygen, and water hardness. A wide variety of physiological and biochemical abnormalities has been reported after fish have been exposed to sublethal concentrations of mercury, although the environmental significance of these effects is difficult to assess. Reproduction is also affected adversely by mercury.

7.4 Toxicity to terrestrial organisms

Plants are generally insensitive to the toxic effects of mercury compounds. Birds fed inorganic mercury show a reduction in food intake and consequent poor growth. Other, more subtle, effects on enzyme systems, cardiovascular function, blood parameters, the immune response, kidney function and structure, and behaviour have been reported. Organomercury compounds are more toxic for birds than are inorganic.

7.5 Effects of mercury in the field

Pollution of the sea with organomercury led to the death of fish and fish-eating birds in Japan. Except for this incident at Minamata, few follow-up studies of the effects of localized release have been conducted. The use of organomercury fungicides as seed dressings in Europe led to the deaths of large numbers of granivorous birds, together with birds of prey feeding on the corpses. Residues of mercury in birds' eggs have been associated with deaths of embryos in shell. The presence of organochlorine residues in the same birds and their eggs makes an accurate assessment of the effects of mercury difficult. It is, however, thought to be a contributing factor in the population decline of some species of raptors.

8. EFFECTS ON EXPERIMENTAL ANIMALS AND *IN VITRO* TEST SYSTEMS

8.1 Single and short-term exposure

Ashe et al. (1953) reported evidence of damage to brain, kidney, heart, and lungs in rabbits exposed acutely to metallic mercury vapour at a mercury concentration of 29 mg/m^3 of air.

The LD_{50} for inorganic mercury, as well as for a number of organomercurials (e.g., arylmercury, alkoxyalkyl- and alkylmercury compounds), lies between 10 and 40 mg/kg body weight for all compounds tested. For mercuric chloride, a value of about 10 mg/kg body weight has been observed after parenteral administration to mice. The similarity in LD_{50} values for these various types of mercury compounds is considered to result from the fact that, when given in acute massive doses, mercury in any chemical form will denature proteins, inactivate enzymes, and cause severe disruption of any tissue with which it comes into contact in sufficient concentrations. The features of acute toxicity usually consist of shock, cardiovascular collapse, acute renal failure, and severe gastrointestinal damage.

8.2 Long-term exposure

8.2.1 *General effects*

WHO (1976), in evaluating a number of experimental studies on animals, concluded that both reversible and irreversible toxic effects may be caused by mercury and its compounds. Microscopically detectable changes have been seen in the organs of dogs, rabbits, and rats exposed to concentrations of elemental mercury vapour ranging from about 100 to 30 000 μg/m^3 for different periods of time. Severe damage was noted in kidneys and brains at mercury levels in air of about 900 μg/m^3 after an exposure period of about 12 weeks. After exposure of dogs to 100 μg mercury/m^3, for 7 h/day, 5 days/week over a period of 83 weeks, no microscopically detectable effects were seen, and tests revealed no abnormalities in kidney function.

In two studies (Fukuda, 1971; Kishi et al., 1978), tremor and behavioural effects were observed in rabbits and rats after several weeks of exposure to metallic mercury vapour at levels of several mg/m^3, although there were no morphological changes in the brain. The symptoms were associated with brain mercury concentrations of about 1 and 20 mg/kg wet weight in the two studies.

8.2.2 Immunological effects

During the last 10-20 years, great attention has been paid to effects of inorganic mercury on the immune system. An important conclusion is that, depending upon the animal strain tested, either auto-immunity or immunosuppression is observed.

8.2.2.1 Auto-immunity

Bariety et al. (1971) showed that about 30% of outbred Wistar rats exposed to mercuric chloride (1.5 or 2.5 mg/kg body weight) 3 times per week for periods of several months developed a membranous glomerulopathy characterized by granular, subepithelial deposits of IgG and C$_3$.

In Brown Norway rats (Sapin et al., 1977; Druet et al., 1978) and in New Zealand rabbits (Roman-Franco et al., 1978) injected with 1 or 2 mg/kg body weight, a systemic auto-immune disease was observed. It appeared in 100% of the rats tested. This disease is characterized by the production of auto-antibodies to renal and extra-renal basement membranes. These antibodies are specific for laminin, type IV collagen, and entactin (Bellon et al., 1982; Fukatsu et al., 1987) and are found deposited along the glomerular basement membrane in a linear pattern. After 3 to 4 weeks, a typical membranous glomerulopathy with granular, subepithelial IgG deposits is observed. The majority of rats develop proteinuria, which progresses in some animals to the nephrotic syndrome (Druet et al., 1978). About half of those with this syndrome die. However, the remainder recover since the disease is transient. Dermatitis and Sjogren's syndrome have been recently detected in Brown Norway rats injected with mercuric chloride (Aten et al., 1988). Contact sensitization to mercury has also been reported to occur in susceptible strains of guinea-pigs (Polak et al., 1968). Auto-immunity in Brown Norway rats appears in the context of a polyclonal activation of B cells. There is a lymphoproliferation (increase in the number of CD4+ T cells and B cells) and hyperimmunoglobulinaemia affecting mainly IgE (Prouvost-Danon et al., 1981; Hirsch et al., 1982; Pelletier et al., 1988a), and several auto-antibodies such as antinuclear antibodies (Hirsch et al., 1982) are produced. All these manifestations are transient. They appear from day 8 following the injection, peak during the third week, and then progressively decline.

A number of other studies have been carried out using Brown Norway rats. Low doses of mercuric chloride (50 μg/kg body weight given 3 times per week) induced auto-immune glomerulopathy, while 100 μg/kg body weight (also 3 times per week) induced both auto-immune glomerulopathy and proteinuria. Mercuric chloride was also effective when given by inhalation (aerosol or intratracheal instillation) or ingestion (Bernaudin et al., 1981; Andres, 1984; Knoflach et al., 1986). Other inorganic mercury compounds, e.g., mercurous chloride given orally or $HgNH_2Cl$-containing ointments, also induce auto-immunity (Druet et al., 1981).

Auto-immune disorders including auto-immune glomerulopathy have been described in other strains of rats (Weening et al., 1978; Druet et al., 1982). In susceptible strains of mice, especially those mice carrying the H-2^s haplotype, long-term exposure to mercuric chloride induces extremely high titres of antinucleolar auto-antibodies (Robinson et al., 1986; Mirtscheva et al., 1987). These auto-antibodies and circulating immune complexes (Hultman & Eneström, 1987) are involved in the glomerular IgG deposits found in the mesangium and in the vessel walls of H-2^s mice treated with mercuric chloride (Hultman & Eneström, 1988). Analysis of the fine specificity of the antinucleolar auto-antibodies revealed that at least some of them react with fibrillarin, a component of U3 small nuclear ribonucleoprotein. Sera from human patients with idiopathic scleroderma contain auto-antibodies with exactly the same specificity (Reuter et al., 1989).

8.2.2.2 Genetics

Rats with certain major histocompatibility haplotypes, such as Lewis rats, are resistant whatever the dose used, while other strains are susceptible (Table 3). The susceptibility of segregants obtained by crossing Brown Norway and Lewis rats has been extensively studied (Druet et al., 1977, 1982; Sapin et al., 1984). It has been demonstrated that susceptibility depends upon 3 or 4 genes. One of them is located within the major histocompatibility complex. Both the major histocompatibility complex-linked and -unlinked genes are required for these auto-immune abnormalities to occur.

Table 3. Susceptibility of various strains of rats to auto-immune glomerulonephritis induced by mercuric chloride

Strain	RT-1 haplotype[a]	Auto-immune glomerulonephritis
BN	n	anti-GBM[b]; MGP[c]
LEW, F/344	l	none
BS, AS, BD IX	l	none
BN-1L[d]	l	none
LEW-1N[d]	n	none
PVG/c, AUG	c	glomerular granular deposits
DA, AVN	a	glomerular granular deposits
AS_2	f	glomerular granular deposits
OKA	k	glomerular granular deposits
BUF	b	glomerular granular deposits
BD V	d	glomerular granular deposits
WAG, LOU	u	none
Wistar Furth	u	MGP

[a] Major histocompatibility complex in the rat.
[b] Antiglomerular basement membrane antibodies.
[c] Membranous glomerulopathy.
[d] Congenic rats with the l RT-1 haplotype on the BN background (BN-1L) or with the n haplotype on the LEW background (LEW-1N).

8.2.2.3 Mechanisms of induction

Mechanisms of induction have been thoroughly studied in rats. Mercuric chloride induces in Brown Norway rats a polyclonal activation of B cells (Hirsch et al., 1982; Pelletier et al., 1988a). T cells are required, since Brown Norway rats with the nude mutation or depleted of T cells are resistant (Pelletier et al., 1987a). It appears that mercuric chloride induces in this rat strain the appearance of T cells able to stimulate class II determinants (also called Ia antigens), which are expressed on the cell membrane of all B cells (Pelletier et al., 1986). The role of such T cells is strongly supported by the fact that T cells from Brown Norway rats injected with mercuric chloride are able to transfer auto-immune manifestations to normal Brown Norway recipients and also to Brown Norway rats depleted of T cells (Pelletier et al., 1988b). This strongly suggests that T cells from rats injected with mercuric chloride are able to stimulate B cells directly. The autoreactive, anticlass II, T cells which recognize normal B cells as well as B cells from rats injected with mercuric chloride may have initially been induced following a modification of class II determinants by mercury, as suggested by Gleichmann et al. (1984). It is also possible that mercuric chloride affects CD8+ (suppressor/cytotoxic) T cells, as suggested by Weening et al. (1981).

The fine mechanism of action at the cellular level (see section 8.7) remains to be elucidated.

8.2.2.4 Autoregulation

The auto-immune disease observed in Brown Norway rats is self-regulated. Abnormalities progressively disappear after the third week. It has been shown that CD8+ (suppressor/cytotoxic) T cells are responsible for this effect (Bowman et al., 1984), together with the appearance of auto-anti-idiotypic antibodies (Chalopin & Lockwood, 1984).

8.2.2.5 Immunosuppression

Lewis rats do not develop auto-immune disorders when injected with mercuric chloride. In contrast, CD8+ (suppressor/cytotoxic) T cells proliferate in the spleen and in the lymph nodes of such animals. As a consequence they develop a non-antigen-specific immunosuppression

(Pelletier et al., 1987c). They do not respond either to classical mitogens or to allo-antigens. More interestingly, mercuric chloride is able to inhibit the development of organ-specific auto-immune disorders such as Heymann's nephritis (Pelletier et al., 1987b) and experimental allergic encephalomyelitis (Pelletier et al., 1988c). The mechanisms are not yet understood.

The mercury model represents a unique tool for evaluating the relationship between genetic and chemically induced immune disregulation.

8.2.2.6 Conclusions

It may be concluded that the most sensitive adverse effect caused by mercuric mercury is the formation of mercuric-mercury-induced auto-immune glomerulonephritis, the first step being the production and deposition of IgG antibodies to the glomerular basement membrane. The Brown Norway rat is a good test species for the study of mercuric-mercury-induced auto-immune glomerulonephritis, although this effect has also been observed in rabbits. Table 4 presents the available studies on auto-immune glomerulonephritis. The lowest-observed-adverse-effect level found in these studies was 16 mg/kg per day via the subcutaneous route of exposure.

8.3 Reproduction, embryotoxicity, and teratogenicity

8.3.1 Males

Very little information on male reproductive effects is available. Lee & Dixon (1975) injected male mice with single doses of mercuric chloride (1 mg mercury/kg body weight) and found a significant decrease in fertility, compared with controls, in controlled mating tests. Normal fertility was restored after about 2 months. In studies by Chowdhury et al. (1986), gradual alterations in testicular tissues were noted in rats treated with mercuric chloride at intraperitoneal dosages of 0.05 mg/kg and 0.1 mg/kg body weight over a period of 90 days. There was a decrease in seminiferous tubular diameter, spermatogenic cell counts, and Leydig cell nuclear diameter, compared with controls.

Table 4. Auto-immune effects of mercuric mercury on the glomerular basement membrane

Animal	Route	Duration	Adverse effect level (mg/kg per day)	Reference
Brown Norway rat	oral	60 days	320	Bernaudin et al. (1981)
Brown Norway rat	oral	60 days	630	Andres (1984)
Brown Norway rat	subcutaneous	12 weeks	16	Druet et al. (1977)
Brown Norway rat	subcutaneous	8 weeks	32[a]	Druet et al. (1978)
Rabbit	intramuscular	1-17 weeks	633	Roman-Franco et al. (1978)

[a] Proteinuria was observed, in addition to the auto-immune glomerulonephritis, in these rats.

8.3.2 Females

Lamperti & Printz (1973) injected female hamsters with daily doses of 1 mg mercuric chloride (8-11 mg mercury/kg) throughout one 4-day estrous cycle (the LD_{50} being 18 mg mercury/kg body weight). There were effects on the reproductive system, including morphological changes of corpora lutea and inhibition of follicular maturation. In further studies (Lamperti & Printz, 1974), it was reported that 60% of female hamsters did not ovulate by day one of the third estrous cycle after having been given a total of 3-4 mg mercuric chloride during the first estrous cycle. Watanabe et al. (1982) injected female hamsters with mercuric chloride at high doses (6.4 or 12.8 mg mercury/kg body weight) during day one of the estrous cycle and observed an inhibition of ovulation. Lamperti & Niewenhuis (1976) injected female hamsters with 1 mg mercuric chloride per day during one estrous cycle and found significantly higher levels of follicle-stimulating hormone in the pituitary gland, compared with controls.

Several investigators have reported abortions following exposure to elemental mercury vapour or inorganic mercury compounds several days after implantation. There are also reports of decreased fetal weight and malformations. Gale & Ferm (1971) injected three groups of female hamsters with a single dose of 2, 3, or 4 mg mercuric acetate (about 1.3-2.5 mg mercury) intravenously on day 8 of gestation. The exposed groups showed resorption frequencies of 12, 34, and 52%, respectively, compared to 4% in the controls. The mothers showed signs of mercury intoxication in the form of weight loss, kidney lesions, and diarrhoea. In later studies (Gale, 1980, 1981), a single injection of mercuric acetate (15 mg/kg body weight) to hamsters produced a cluster of cardiac and non-cardiac abnormalities. The most important aspects of embryotoxicity were resorptions, retardation, and abnormal heart. Significant but varied interstrain differences were observed. Holt & Webb (1986) exposed pregnant Wistar rats intravenously to mercuric chloride at different periods of gestation. During mid-gestation the minimum effective teratogenic dose of mercury (0.79 mg/kg total body weight) was high in relation to the maternal LD_{50} and the incidence of fetal malformations, mainly brain defects, was

23% in all live fetuses. In rats of different gestational ages, uptake of Hg^{2+} by the fetus at this dose level decreased sharply between day 12 and day 13. The teratogenic effects on the fetus and damage to the maternal kidneys, however, were essentially the same in animals dosed with Hg^{2+} either immediately before or immediately after these gestational ages. The authors considered it probable, therefore, that fetal defects resulted not from any direct action of Hg^{2+} on the conceptuses but either from the inhibition of the transport of essential metabolites from the mother or from maternal kidney dysfunction.

In a study by Rizzo & Furst (1972), three groups of female rats were exposed to single oral doses of mercuric oxide equivalent to 2 mg mercury/dose. Each dose of mercury was given suspended in 2 ml peanut oil. The three groups received the mercury on day 5, 12, or 19 after conception. External malformations were observed in 29.7%, 6.8%, and 3.4% of cases, respectively, while the three control groups had values between 0 and 2%. The two observable effects that mercury had on rat fetuses were arrest of general growth, as indicated by the number of runts, and inhibition of eye formation. The mothers showed no effects from the treatment. The data, if confirmed, are of particular interest, as mercuric oxide is fairly insoluble.

Steffek et al. (1987) reported the effects of elemental mercury vapour exposure on pregnant Sprague-Dawley rats. The rats were exposed to elemental mercury vapour at concentrations of 100, 500, or 1000 $\mu g/m^3$ during the entire gestational period (chronic exposure) or during the period of organogenesis (days 10-15, acute exposure). Macroscopic examination of fetuses obtained from pregnant rats exposed acutely or chronically to 100 $\mu g/m^3$ revealed no increased incidence of congenital malformations or resorptions when compared to room or chamber controls. However, acute exposure to 500 $\mu g/m^3$ resulted in an increase in the number of resorptions (5/41), and chronic exposure at this concentration resulted in two fetuses (out of 84 that were examined) with cranial defects. There were also single cases of encephalomeningocoele, dome-shaped cranial configuration, and cleft palate (Steffek, A.J., written personal communication to the American

Dental Association). Acute exposure at 1000 $\mu g/m^3$ resulted in an increase in the rate of resorptions (8/71), and chronic exposure at this dose level produced a decrease in maternal and fetal weights, relative to the control groups, and an increase in the number of resorptions (7/28).

8.4 Mutagenicity and related end-points

Mercuric mercury affects the mitotic spindle in plants, which may lead to an abnormal distribution of chromosomes (Ramel, 1972; Leonard et al., 1983). It is not a potent inducer of dominant lethal mutations in mice (Suter, 1975). Zasukhina et al. (1983) reported the induction of single-stranded DNA breaks after exposure of cultures of mice embryo cells to mercury chloride. The mercury did not induce mutations but had a strong lethal effect in a survival test of vaccinia virus. A shortening of the chromosome length in human lymphocytes exposed *in vitro* has been observed (Andersen et al., 1983). Mercuric mercury did not induce chromosomal aberrations in human lymphocytes and in mammalian cells *in vitro* (Paton & Allison 1972; Umeda & Nishimura, 1979). Positive results in the recombination assay with mercuric chloride have been reported by Kanematsu et al. (1980). Effects have been reported on DNA repair in mammalian cells (Robison et al., 1984). There was an increase in C-mitotic figures and segregational errors in human lymphocytes and in Indian muntjac fibroblasts (Verschaeve et al., 1984, 1985). Based on studies of *Drosophila melanogaster,* Magnusson & Ramel (1986) found a pronounced variation in tolerance between 12 wild type strains when testing a number of metal compounds, including mercuric chloride. Morimoto et al. (1982) reported that in human whole blood cultures selenite prevents the induction of sister-chromatid exchanges by mercuric chloride.

The US Agency for Toxic Substances and Disease Registry (ATSDR, 1989) has reviewed several *in vitro* genotoxicity studies on mercury compounds. Mercuric chloride was found to induce gene mutations in mouse lymphoma cells (Oberly et al., 1982) and DNA damage in rat and mouse fibroblasts (Zasukhina et al., 1983). It was observed to bind to rat fibroblast chromatin (Rozalski & Wierzbicki,

1983; Christie et al., 1986). Using the alkaline elution assay in intact Chinese hamster ovary cells, several studies have shown that mercuric chloride can cause single-strand breaks in DNA (Cantoni et al., 1982, 1984a, 1984b; Cantoni & Costa, 1983; Christie et al., 1984, 1986). Furthermore, Cantoni & Costa (1983) found that the DNA-damaging effect of mercuric chloride is enhanced by a concurrent inhibitory effect that mercury has on DNA repair mechanisms.

8.5 Carcinogenicity

WHO (1976) reported no evidence that inorganic mercury is carcinogenic. In a study by Schroeder & Mitchener (1975), groups of mice were exposed to various metals, including mercuric chloride. After a lifetime of exposure to 5 μg mercury/litre in basal drinking-water, 51.2% (21 out of 41) of the mice revealed tumours compared to 29.8% (14 out of 47) among controls. The incidence was higher than for any of the other metals tested, but the authors concluded that no element was significantly tumorigenic. Mercury has not been reviewed by IARC (IARC, 1987). The US EPA (1989) has classified inorganic mercury as a group O compound, i.e. it is not classifiable as to human carcinogenicity.

8.6 Factors modifying toxicity

Factors such as age, sex, nutritional state, and oral exposure giving rise to sensitization are likely to affect the relationship between dose and effect or response. The type of chemical exposure (whether to elemental mercury or to mercuric mercury salts) is an important determinant for the toxic effect and to differences in distribution.

As described in section 6.1.2, Kostial et al. (1978) observed a high degree of absorption of inorganic mercury in newborn rats after oral exposure to mercuric chloride. The immature rodent kidney is, on the other hand, less sensitive to mercury exposure than the adult kidney, as less accumulation takes place in the kidney of the newborn pups (Daston et al., 1983). No information is available concerning age effects in humans.

Exposure of rats to high concentrations of mercury vapour induced metallothionein in kidney tissue that resulted in the binding of divalent mercury (Sapota et al., 1974). Female rats are less susceptible than male rats to the nephrotoxic effect of mercuric mercury (Magos et al., 1974). This seems to be related to the metallothionein content of the kidney, which is higher in females and is increased by estradiol treatment (Nishiyama et al., 1987). Administration of zinc to rats reduced the renal toxic effects of mercuric mercury and induced an increase in the glutathione (Fukino et al., 1986) and metallothionein content of renal tissue (Yoshikawa & Ohta, 1982). Zinc treatment in hamsters injected with mercuric salt reduced the embryotoxic and teratogenic effects produced by treatment with the mercuric salt alone (Gale, 1984).

Selenium has been found to affect the distribution of mercuric mercury in rats (Parizek & Ostadalova, 1967; Nygaard & Hansen, 1978), mice (Eybl et al., 1969), rabbits (Imura & Naganuma, 1978; Naganuma & Imura, 1980), and pigs (Hansen et al., 1981). As a consequence of this redistribution, a decrease in toxicity has also been observed (Parizek & Ostadalova, 1967; Johnson & Pond, 1974). Mercury forms a mercury-protein complex with selenium (Burk et al., 1974), which can be identified in plasma and blood cells (Chen et al., 1974; Imura & Naganuma, 1978). When given with selenium, mercury is retained longer in blood and, as a consequence, accumulation in the kidney is decreased. Mercury taken up by the kidney is bound to a protein-selenium complex, and, on administration of equivalent amounts of selenium, the binding to metallothionein is diminished and may be negligible (Komsta-Szumska & Chmielnicka, 1977; Mengel & Karlog, 1980). A consequence of the changed binding of mercury in blood brought about by selenium is that transport of selenium and mercury through the placenta membranes is inhibited (Parizek et al., 1971).

So far only selenate or selenite compounds, and not the naturally occurring selenium compounds in food, have been studied in detail. However, Magos et al. (1984, 1987) compared the distribution and form of mercury and protection against the nephrotoxic effects of mercury after exposure to different forms or compounds of selenium. It was concluded that dietary selenium is less efficient than selenite as an antidote against mercurial nephrotoxicity.

Studies of selenium interaction with mercuric mercury have mainly been carried out in rodents. Selenium metabolism in humans is different from that in most animals, and selenium dependency in humans is comparatively less than that in rodents. However, observations in workers exposed to mercury vapour indicate that there is also a selenium-mercury interaction in humans. Selenium and mercury concentrations with a molar ratio of 1:1 have been found in organs such as the brain, thyroid, and pituitary (Kosta et al., 1975; Rossi et al., 1976). In renal biopsies from two mercury-intoxicated patients, inclusion bodies were seen in lysosomes of renal tubules, and it was demonstrated that these inclusion bodies contained selenium and mercury (Aoi et al., 1985). In 28 workers exposed to mercury vapour, the selenium excretion in urine was high compared to non-exposed workers (Alexander et al., 1983). However, this was not confirmed by Suzuki et al. (1986), who studied 57 workers exposed to mercury vapour. They found a decrease in selenium excretion as mercury excretion in the urine increased.

As discussed in section 6.2, ethanol inhibits the enzyme catalase, which is the main enzyme responsible for the oxidation of mercury in blood and tissues. Ethanol consumption thus modifies the balance between oxidation and reduction of mercury in tissues. As a consequence, less mercury vapour is absorbed from the lungs, more mercury exists unoxidized in the blood, and more mercury is transported to the brain. It is unclear whether the observed decrease of mercury in the brain is due to the fact that less mercury is oxidized and retained in the brain or that more retained mercury is lost from the brain as a result of reduction following the intake of ethanol. The mercury content of the brain following acute exposure to mercury in acatalasaemic mice is greater than that of mercury-exposed control mice (Ogata et al., 1987). This is also the case with the fetal brain after exposure of pregnant female acatalasaemic mice (Ogata & Meguro, 1986).

8.7 Mechanisms of toxicity - mode of action

The neurotoxic effect seen after exposure to metallic mercury vapour is attributable to the divalent mercury ion formed through oxidation in the brain tissue. Interference with enzyme function by binding to sulfhydryl groups is one possible mechanism. Kark (1979) reviewed the available evidence regarding the inhibitory effect of mercuric ions on different enzyme systems (in vitro and in vivo). Mercury concentrations at which enzyme inhibition appears are consistent with concentrations at which toxic effects on the central nervous system are observed. The in vivo conditions are, however, complicated. Ligands capable of binding mercuric ions, e.g., sulfhydryl groups and selenohydrol groups, are ubiquitous and associated with proteins. These ligands may have a protective or scavenging effect, thereby preventing interference with important receptors. Mercuric ions penetrate cell membranes to a very limited degree. In contrast mercury vapour penetrates more readily due to its lipophilicity. Miyamoto (1983) demonstrated with frog nerve-muscle preparations that mercuric mercury penetrates the nerve cell membrane through sodium and calcium channels, causing an irreversible depolarization and an increase in transmitter release. There is a subsequent irreversible block of transmitter release. Transport through the cell membrane via the formation of carrier complexes would also be a possibility, although this has not been demonstrated. Mercury has been found intracellularly in nerve cells after exposure to mercury vapour (Cassano et al., 1966) and also after prolonged exposure to mercuric chloride in the rat (Moller-Madsen & Danscher, 1986).

Mercuric ions react with DNA and RNA in vitro and may change the tertiary structure of these molecules (Eichhorn & Clark, 1963; Gruenwedel & Davidson, 1966). Inhibition of protein synthesis has been observed in cell systems as well as in cell-free systems at a mercury concentration equivalent to 2×10^{-5} mol/litre (Nakada et al., 1980). Similar mercury concentrations have been observed to increase the pre-synaptic release of the transmitter substance acetylcholine (Kostial & Landeka, 1975; Manalis & Cooper, 1975). An increase in the release of dopamine in the rat brain after treatment with mercury (10^{-5} mol per litre) at a level of 2 μg/g was observed by Bondy et al. (1979).

Mercury may interfere with membrane structure in vitro by hydrolysing specific lipids (Ganser & Kirschner, 1985), causing membrane lesions, and by reducing lipid synthesis in nerve cells (Cloez et al., 1987). Furthermore, an irreversible interference with the post-synaptic membrane has been observed (Manalis & Cooper, 1975; Juang, 1976).

Knowledge regarding the mechanism of mercury neurotoxicity, following exposure to mercury vapour, is still fragmentary. Little data has so far emerged concerning morphological changes in the human or primate brain. Mercury has been demonstrated in rats within the motor nuclei of the rhombencephalon and the cerebral cortex, the highest concentrations occurring in striated areas and within the deep nuclei of the cerebellum. A proportionately high level was seen in the anterior horn motor neurones of the spinal cord. The localization was generally interneuronal, but was also seen in the cytoplasm of glial and ependymal cells (Moller-Madsen & Danscher, 1986). In human cases of mercury poisoning, chromatolysis in scattered neurones was observed in the occipital lobe of the brain and there was a loss of Purkinje cells (Takahata et al., 1970). Davis et al. (1974) demonstrated, in two human cases, mercury in the cytoplasm of neurones in the nuclei olivaris and dentatus, in Purkinje cells, in anterior horn cells of the spinal cord, and in the neurones of the substantia nigra. In both cases a decrease in the number of neurones of the granular cell layer in the cerebellum and, possibly, also of Purkinje cells was seen.

The mechanism behind the nephrotoxic effect of inorganic mercury is discussed in sections 8.2 and 9.3. Here it can be summarized that two types of renal injury have been observed. The first is a glomerular injury caused by an auto-immune reaction induced by mercury and resulting in antibody formation against the glomerular tissue, deposition of immune complex, glomerular nephritis, proteinuria, and nephrotic syndrome. Alternatively, immune complexes containing other mercury-induced anti-bodies may be deposited in the glomeruli. The second is a renal tubular damage affecting the proximal tubules and developing in parallel with the accumulation of mercury in the renal tubular cells. This damage results in a loss of renal tubular enzymes, such as γ-glutamyl transferase, and lysosome enzymes, such as β-galactosidase, β-glucuronidase and N-acetyl-β-glucosaminidase (Foa et al., 1976), and in decreased reabsorption leading to an increased secretion of endogenous trace elements such as zinc and copper (Chmielnicka et al., 1986). An early effect is an inhibition of protein synthesis. A swelling of the endoplasmic reticulum with disaggregation of poly-ribosomes is observed in electron microscopy. Eventually, renal tubular necrosis and renal failure develop (Wessel, 1967; Gritzka & Trump, 1968; Barnes et al., 1980; Pezerovic et al., 1981).

The immunotoxic effect of inorganic mercury is prob-ably the least understood effect of exposure to inorganic mercury. Mercuric mercury has been observed as a potent stimulator of human T lymphocytes *in vitro* (Schöpf et al., 1969; Nordlind & Henze, 1984; Nordlind, 1985). Mercury is initially bound to lymphocyte membranes, but it has also been demonstrated that there is an uptake of mercury by the nuclei (Nordlind, 1985) at levels likely to occur in blood following exposure to mercury vapour. It can be speculated that this phenomenon may be related to the rather generalized syndromes observed in children, such as acrodynia or "Pink disease" (Warkany, 1966; Skerfving & Vostal, 1972) and the rather generalized and unspecific syndromes reported to be related to dental amalgam fill-ings, but with an unproven relation to mercury exposure (section 9.7).

9. EFFECTS ON HUMANS

WHO (1976) dealt primarily with effects of occupational exposure to mercury vapour. Apart from accidental exposure, there was little information on exposure to inorganic mercury among the general population. Recent data indicate that the release of mercury vapour from amalgam fillings may dominate exposure to inorganic mercury among the general population (Elinder et al., 1988; WHO, 1990). Other sources are a fish-rich diet (biotransformation of alkyl mercury present in some species of fish resulting in the accumulation of inorganic mercury), environmental pollution in the vicinity of industrial sources, toxic waste sites, and accidental spillage. Mercury-containing pharmaceuticals may also be significant sources of exposure for some populations.

The present review will focus on possible chronic effects of long-term, low-level occupational exposure and, for the general population, of mercury released from amalgam. However, a brief review of acute effects will be given. In general, the available information is presented according to the effects on organs or organ systems. Sometimes this is not possible, as is the case for the combination of a number of unspecific symptoms that have been associated by some with exposure from dental amalgams. Whenever dose-response relationships are discussed, it should be borne in mind that data on exposure levels in the past are scarce. Quality assurance data are with few exceptions not reported. In most studies personal samplers were not used but only static samplers, which can be a source of considerable error in the estimated absorbed dose, as demonstrated by Stopford et al. (1978) and Roels et al. (1987).

Data related to response rates are sometimes difficult to interpret. The studies are as a rule cross-sectional, and so selection bias, which may lead to either an underestimation or an overestimation of risks, can occur. The numbers of exposed subjects and controls are often small. For quite a few of the parameters studied, the results may be influenced by the investigator and "interviewer bias" is thus possible.

9.1 Acute toxicity

Workers acutely exposed (4-8 h) to calculated elemental mercury levels of 1.1 to 44 mg/m^3 due to an accident exhibited chest pains, dyspnoea, cough, haemoptysis, impairment of pulmonary function, and evidence of interstitial pneumonitis (McFarland & Reigel, 1978). Acute mercury poisoning with mercurial pneumonitis was reported among four men after they were exposed to mercury vapour while attempting home gold ore purification using a gold-mercury amalgam and sulfuric acid (Levin et al., 1988). Urine mercury levels were 169 to 520 µg/litre in two cases. Probably there was also substantial exposure to sulfur dioxide and sulfuric acid.

Troen et al. (1951) reported 18 cases of human poisoning following oral ingestion of single doses of mercuric chloride, nine of which resulted in death. The lethal doses ranged from 29 mg/kg body weight to at least 50 mg/kg. The most common autopsy findings in these cases were gastrointestinal lesions (ranging from mild gastritis to severe necrotizing ulceration of the mucosa) and renal lesions that had resulted in renal failure.

9.2 Effects on the nervous system

Most information focuses on effects on the central nervous system following occupational exposure. The central nervous system is the critical organ for mercury vapour exposure (WHO, 1976). Acute exposure has given rise to psychotic reactions characterized by delirium, hallucinations, and suicidal tendency. Occupational exposure has resulted in erethism, with irritability, excitability, excessive shyness, and insomnia as the principal features of a broad-ranging functional disturbance. With continuing exposure, a fine tremor develops, initially involving the hands and later spreading to the eyelids, lips, and tongue, causing violent muscular spasms in the most severe cases. The tremor is reflected in the handwriting which has a characteristic appearance. In milder cases, erethism and tremor regress slowly over a period of years following removal from exposure. Decreased nerve conduction velocity in mercury-exposed workers has been demonstrated (Bidstrup et al., 1951). Long-term, low-level exposure has been found to be associated with less pronounced symptoms of erethism, characterized by fatigue, irritability, loss of memory, vivid dreams, and depression (WHO, 1976).

9.2.1 Relations between mercury in the central nervous system and effects/response

There is very little information on brain mercury levels in cases of mercury poisoning, and nothing that makes it possible to estimate a no-observed-effect level or a dose-response curve. Furthermore, the available data are uncertain as they are not accompanied by analytical quality control information.

Brigatti (1949) reported mercury concentrations of 6-9 mg/kg in the brain of two workers exposed to mercury vapour and with signs of mercury poisoning 2 years before they died. In two similar cases, Takahata et al. (1970) reported 5-34 mg mercury/kg in different parts of the brain. In two fatal cases of poisoning, which followed many years of exposure to high doses of calomel as a laxative, mercury concentrations of about 4 mg/kg in the frontal lobe cortex were reported, and in one of the cases a concentration of 106 mg/kg was found in the inferior olive (Davis et al., 1974; Wands et al., 1974). The symptoms were dementia, erethism, colitis, and renal failure. A dose of two tablet laxatives, each containing 120 mg of USP-grade mercurous chloride, had been taken daily for 25 years in one case and for 6 years in the other.

9.2.2 Relations between mercury in air, urine or blood and effects/response

9.2.2.1 Occupational exposure

WHO (1976) found no evidence of the classical symptoms of mercurialism, erethism, intentional tremor, or gingivitis below a time-weighted occupational exposure to mercury in air of 100 μg/m^3. A report on cottage industry mercury smelting in China (Wu et al., 1989) has confirmed the classical symptoms at exposure levels of up to 600 μg/m^3. Symptoms such as loss of appetite and psychological disturbance have also been found to occur at mercury levels below 100 μg/m^3 (WHO, 1976).

Zeglio (1958) observed that following cessation of exposure, symptoms and signs of neurological impairment regress slowly in the milder cases of poisoning affecting the nervous system. However, in the more severe cases, neurological impairment persists and may become exacerbated.

One of the studies on which WHO (1976) based its conclusions was carried out by Smith et al. (1970). This study covered the prevalence of several medical findings in 567 workers in a number of chloralkali factories in the USA in relation to mercury vapour exposure (Fig. 6). The authors concluded that the data showed no significant signs or symptoms in persons exposed to mercury vapour at or below a level of 0.1 mg/m^3. Subjective symptoms appeared to increase at lower exposure levels, but the authors questioned this finding because of the confounding effect of alcohol. In a follow-up of part of this study, Bunn et al. (1986) did not find significant differences in the frequency of objective or subjective findings related to mercury exposure, which generally was said to range from 50 to 100 μg/m^3 (time-weighted average). The report, however, did not give sufficient information about several methodological questions, including quality assurance aspects and possible confounding variables.

Later studies, covering industries where exposure has been high, have pointed towards the importance of urine mercury peaks in excess of 500 μg/litre for the development of neurological signs and symptoms (Langolf et al., 1978, 1981). Urine mercury peaks in excess of 100 μg per litre have been associated with impaired performance in mechanical and visual memory tasks and psychomotor ability tests (Forzi et al., 1976).

There is also a report (Albers et al., 1988) that, as long as 20 to 35 years after exposure, subjects who had experienced urine mercury peak levels above 600 μg per litre demonstrated significantly decreased strength, decreased coordination, increased tremor, decreased sensation, and increased prevalence of Babinski and snout reflexes when compared with control subjects. Furthermore, subjects with reported clinical polyneuropathy had significantly higher peak levels of mercury in urine than the subjects without those signs. The reported signs of the

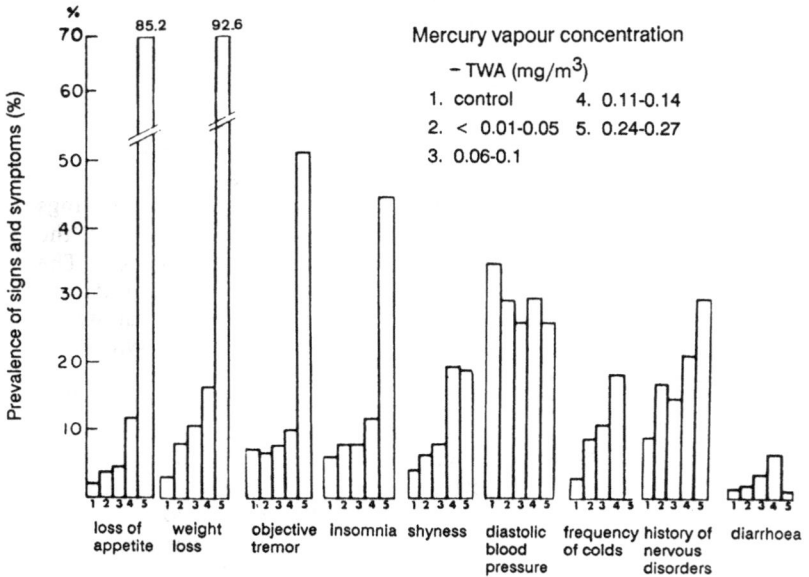

Fig. 6. Relation between mercury in work room and certain signs and symptoms (From: Smith et al., 1970).

presence of an upper motor neuron lesion will require further investigation. Many measures demonstrating significant differences between exposed and unexposed subjects were age dependant, but a multiple regression analysis showed that the association between neurological signs and mercury exposure remained after allowing for age (Albers et al., 1988).

Several reports address studies where the investigators have looked into possible effects at much lower exposure levels. In a study of 142 exposed and 65 control subjects, Miller et al. (1975) examined subclinical effects related to exposure to inorganic mercury in the chloralkali industry and in a factory for the manufacture of magnetic materials. Mercury levels in urine varied from normal to over 1000 μg/litre. Neurological examination found evidence of eyelid fasciculation, hyperactive deep tendon reflexes and dermatographia, but these findings did not correlate with urinary mercury levels or length of exposure. However, a power spectral analysis of forearm tremor, by which it was possible to quantify tremor frequency distribution and amplitude, showed a significant increase in average tremor frequency with elevated urinary mercury level. An effect was observed at urine concentrations above about 50 μg/litre.

Roels et al. (1982) studied psychomotor performance in workers in a chloralkali plant and a factory for the manufacture of electric batteries. The results suggested that preclinical psychomotor dysfunction related to the central nervous system occurs when blood mercury levels rise to values between 10 and 20 μg/litre and when mercury in urine exceeds 50 μg/g creatinine. However, even in a subgroup with urinary mercury levels below 50 μg/g creatinine, some parameters differed from those of a control group.

In a further study, Roels et al. (1985) examined 131 male workers and 54 female workers exposed to metallic mercury vapour in various Belgian factories. The controls used were 114 non-exposed male workers and 48 female workers. The subjects in the control and exposed groups were closely matched with respect to age, weight, and height. Also several other confounding factors were kept under control. One criterion for the inclusion of exposed workers was that they should have been uninterruptedly exposed to mercury vapour for at least 1 year prior to the study. A large number of questions were asked in order to detect symptoms mainly related to nervous system disturbances. A self-administered questionnaire, which was completed the next day by the examiner, was the basis for this information. A large number of CNS tests were used, such as reaction time, flicker fusion, colour discrimination, short-term memory, and hand tremor. Mercury was measured in urine and blood. Renal function was studied using various tests, including total protein and β-2-microglobulin in blood and urine, and retinol-binding protein, albumin, and the lysosomal enzyme β-galactosidase in urine. Several symptoms mainly related to the central nervous system (memory disturbances, depressive feelings, fatigue, irritability) were more prevalent in the exposed subjects than in the controls. The means and 95 percentiles for urine mercury levels in non-exposed and exposed subjects were, respectively, 52 and 147 μg/g creatinine for males and 37 and 63 μg/g creatinine for females. The symptoms were, however, not related to exposure parameters. The authors therefore considered it possible that the reporting of these symptoms was influenced by knowledge of exposure to mercury vapour. There were no significant disturbances in short-term memory, simple reaction time, critical flicker fusion, and colour discrimination ability that were related to the mercury exposure. However, an effect on hand tremor was observed in males. The prevalence was 5% in the non-exposed group and 15% in the exposed group. Duration of exposure seemed to be more important than exposure intensity, but an increased prevalence of tremor was apparent in both the groups with the lowest exposure (urine mercury level of 5-50 μg/g creatinine) and that with the shortest exposure duration (1-4 years).

Among 26 workers exposed to mercury vapour in a chloralkali plant or in the production of fluorescent tubes and acetaldehyde, there was an increased incidence of reports of hand tremor, compared with a control group (Fawer et al., 1983). The exposure, based on personal air sampling, was on average only 26 μg/m³. The mean urine concentration was 20 μg/g creatinine (11.3 μmol/mol creatinine). Similar results were reported in a study by Verberk et al. (1986), where 21 workers in a fluorescent lamp production factory were examined. The excretion of mercury in urine varied between 15 and 95 μg/g creatinine, the average value being 35 μg/g creatinine. No control group was examined, but with increasing exposure effects were seen in several tremor parameters. The effects were reported to occur irrespective of cigarette or alcohol consumption or age.

Piikivi et al. (1984) reported decreased verbal intelligence and memory in a group of 36 chloralkali workers compared with a control group. Such effects were seen more frequently in a subgroup where the urine mercury level was above 56 μg/litre than in a subgroup where levels were below this value. Piikivi & Hänninen (1989) made refined analyses of the results of another study on 60 chloralkali workers and matched controls. The exposed workers had an average urine mercury concentration of 84.1 nmol/litre. Neither the perceptual-motor, memory, nor learning abilities of the mercury-exposed workers showed any disturbances when compared to the controls. However, the exposed workers reported statistically significantly more disturbances of memory than the controls. According to multivariate analysis of variance, the memory disorders were significantly associated with the form of workshift but not with the level of exposure. In a further study (Piikivi & Tolonen, 1989), EEG changes were found in a group of 40 workers, compared to matched controls, after several years of exposure to an average metallic mercury vapour level of about 25 $\mu g/m^3$ air, corresponding to a urine mercury level of about 20 μg/litre. The EEG was significantly slower and more attenuated in exposed workers.

Results from the studies of Schiele et al. (1979), Triebig et al. (1981), and Triebig & Schaller (1982) indicate effects on cognitive functions and memory. However, it is not possible to draw conclusions concerning dose-response relationships from these studies. In a study by Schuckmann (1979), 39 chloralkali workers with an average urinary mercury concentration of about 100 μg/litre were compared with a control group. There was no evidence of changes in psychomotor activity. Smith et al. (1983) studied effects on short-term memory in one group of 26 male chloralkali workers with an exposure corresponding to urine mercury levels averaging 195 μg/litre and one group of 60 male workers where the average urine mercury level was 108 μg/litre. The severity of the effects was found to be related to the intensity of mercury exposure.

There are some reports (Levine et al., 1982; Shapiro et al., 1982; Singer et al., 1987; Zampollo et al., 1987) that elemental mercury vapour causes peripheral neuropathy at urinary levels of 50-100 μg/litre. Levine et al. (1982) found a dose-response relationship between urine mercury concentrations above 50 μg/litre and nerve conduction tests.

9.2.2.2 *General population exposure*

The exposure of the general population is typically low, but occasionally may be raised to the level of occupational exposure and can even result in adverse health effects. Thus mishandling of liquid mercury, mercury dispersed from jars, broken thermometers, fluorescent lamps, and ingestion of mercury batteries have resulted in severe intoxication and occasionally acute pneumonitis. Children of mercury workers can also be exposed to mercury vapour from contaminated work clothes. Hudson et al. (1987) reported considerable mercury exposure among children of mercury workers from a thermometer plant. The median urine mercury level of 23 workers' children was 25 μg/litre compared with a value of 5 μg/litre among 39 controls. Three of the workers' children had urine mercury levels above 50 μg/litre; one was above 100 μg per litre. Mercury levels in workers' homes had a median value of 0.24 μg/m^3 compared with 0.05 μg/m^3 in non-workers' homes. No signs of mercury intoxication were reported, based on a questionnaire to parents and on a neurological examination that included assessment of tremor by spectral power analysis. Urine protein was measured only by dipstick. The reported air mercury levels do not explain the high urinary concentrations. There must have been exposure from sources that were not identified, e.g., clothes. It is not known what measures were taken to avoid contamination of sampling bottles.

Children who are exposed to mercury vapour from interior latex paint may develop acrodynia. In 1989, a 4-year-old boy developed severe acrodynia 10 days after the inside of his home was painted with 64 litres of interior latex paint containing 945 mg mercury/litre. He sequentially developed leg cramps, a generalized rash, pruritis, sweating, tachycardia, an intermittent low-grade fever, marked personality change, erythema and desquamation of the hands, feet, and nose, weakness of the pelvic and pectoral girdles, and lower extremity nerve dysfunction. The level of mercury in a 24-h collection of urine was 65 μg/litre.

9.3 Effects on the kidney

The kidney is the critical organ following the ingestion of inorganic bivalent mercury salts. Oliguria, anuria, and death from renal failure resulting from acute tubular necrosis has occurred not infrequently in the past following the ingestion of mercuric chloride either accidentally or with suicidal intent, and such cases have also followed therapeutic administration of mercurials. At the other extreme, organic mercurials have until recent years been used extensively in medical practice as effective diuretics in the management of congestive cardiac failure. Occupational exposure to metallic mercury has for long been associated with the development of proteinuria, both in workers with other evidence of mercury poisoning and in those without such evidence. An increased prevalence of proteinuria in mercury workers, compared with a control group, and a significant correlation between urinary mercury excretion and protein excretion have been demonstrated (Joselow & Goldwater, 1967). Less commonly, occupational exposure has been followed by the nephrotic syndrome (Kazantzis et al., 1962). Such cases have also followed the therapeutic administration of mercurials, although the role of mercury in some of these reported cases, where other etiological factors may have been operative, is less clear. Two children developed the nephrotic syndrome following a spillage of mercury in their bedroom from a broken thermometer (Agner & Jans, 1978). The current evidence suggests that the nephrotic syndrome following absorption of mercury compounds results from an immunotoxic response.

9.3.1 Immunological effects

WHO (1976) stated that effects of elemental mercury vapour on the kidney had been reported only at doses higher than those associated with the onset of CNS signs and symptoms. Since then several new studies have been carried out, and kidney effects have been seen at lower exposure levels. Simultaneously, experimental studies on animals have shown that inorganic mercury may induce auto-immune glomerulonephritis in all species tested but not in all strains, indicating a genetic predisposition.

Kazantzis (1978) and Filliastre et al. (1988) reviewed the role of hypersensitivity and the immune response in influencing susceptibility to metal toxicity, and gave evidence of several case histories of clinical kidney disease after exposure to mercury, occupationally as well as among the general population. Of 60 adult African women using skin-lightening creams containing inorganic mercury, 26 developed the nephrotic syndrome (Barr et al., 1972). Kibukamusoke et al. (1974) reported one case of membranous nephropathy, due to the use of skin-lightening cream, where immunofluorescence showed finely granular IgG, IgM, and C3 complement deposits. IgG and C3 complement deposits were reported also by Lindqvist et al. (1974) in eight cases with nephrotic syndrome. The authors also observed similar kidney changes in two rabbits after application (3 times per week for more than three months) of skin-lightening cream to the skin area between the ears. The rabbits developed proteinuria and died.

9.3.2 Relations between mercury in organs and effects/response

Only very limited information is available. In the report by Davis et al. (1974) referred to in section 9.1.1, kidney mercury concentrations of 422 mg/kg and 25 mg/kg were measured in two fatal cases of poisoning. However, no information was given on whether or not adverse effects on the kidney were observed.

9.3.3 Relations between mercury in air, urine and/or blood and effect/response

Foa et al. (1976) examined chloralkali industry workers exposed to mercury vapour concentrations of 0.06 to 0.3 mg/m^3. There were 15 cases of glomerular proteinuria among 81 workers examined. Increased levels of certain lysosomal enzymes were found in plasma, and this effect was observed even in a group where the average urine mercury level was only 35 μg/litre.

Stewart et al. (1977) examined 21 laboratory assistants exposed not only to metallic mercury vapour but also to mercuric mercury and formaldehyde and found increased urinary excretion of protein. Air concentrations of mercury were 10-50 μg/m^3, and the median urine mercury excretion rate was 53 μg/24 h (about 35 μg/litre urine). Preventive measures were taken and in a follow-up study of nine subjects one year later there was no evidence of proteinuria.

Buchet et al. (1980) examined a group of 63 workers in a chloralkali plant and found, compared with a control group, increased plasma and urinary concentrations of the enzyme β-galactosidase, increased urinary excretion of proteins with high relative molecular mass, and slightly increased β-2-microglobulin concentration in the plasma without a concomitant increase in urinary concentration. The urinary excretion of transferrin, albumin, and β-galactosidase was significantly correlated with the urine concentration of mercury. The likelihood of finding effects increased in workers with urine and/or blood mercury concentrations of over 50 μg/g creatinine or 30 μg/litre blood. The data indicated an increased concentration of β-galactosidase even in the group of workers with an average urine mercury concentration of about 20 μg/g creatinine. According to the authors the results suggest that mercury vapour exposure may lead to a slight glomerular dysfunction in some workers, and their hypothesis is that the glomerular dysfunction is a result of an auto-immune reaction.

The same research group (Roels et al., 1982) studied the prevalence of proteinuria among 43 workers exposed to metallic mercury vapour (median urine and blood mercury levels of 71 μg/g creatinine and 21 μg/litre, respectively) in two other factories (section 9.2.2). Increased total proteinuria and albuminuria was slightly more prevalent in the mercury-exposed group than in the control group.

No evidence of renal dysfunction (proteinuria, albuminuria, retinol-binding proteins, aminoaciduria, creatinine, and β-2-microglobulin in serum) was found among 62 exposed workers in a chloralkali plant and a zinc-mercury amalgam factory, compared with a control group (Lauwerys et al., 1983). The mean urine mercury concentration in the exposed group was 56 μg/g creatinine. In eight exposed workers, but in none of the controls, antibodies against laminin, a non-collagen glycoprotein in the glomerular basal membrane, were found. However, in a later study of workers in another chloralkali plant and in a battery factory (Bernard et al., 1987), the prevalence of circulating anti-laminin antibodies was not increased.

Stonard et al. (1983) examined a group of about 100 chloralkali industry workers with an average urine mercury level of 67 μg/g creatinine. They found no evidence of renal dysfunction and no increased excretion of proteins. An increase in circulating immune complexes was found but there were no anti-glomerular basement membrane antibodies in the serum.

Roels et al. (1985) examined the renal function of 185 workers exposed to metallic mercury vapour (see also section 9.2.2.1). Slight tubular effects were detected in both male and female workers, in the form of an increased urinary β-galactosidase activity and an increased urinary excretion of retinol-binding proteins. The effects were dose related. Some increase in the prevalence of abnormal values was seen even at mean urine mercury levels of about 30 μg/g creatinine. However, there was not, as was the case for tremor, a dose-response relationship concerning the length of the exposure period.

Rosenman et al. (1986) reported that urinary N-acetyl-β-glucosaminidase (NAG) enzyme levels increased with increasing urine mercury levels over the range of 100-250 μg/litre. In a study of chloralkali industry workers, there was a slight increase in the urine NAG concentration among exposed workers (average urine mercury level of 50 μg/litre), compared with a control group (Langworth, 1987).

Another way of studying kidney effects is to measure the brush-border protein (BB-50) concentration in the urine. This indicates the loss of organic tissue rather than functional changes in the kidney cells. The urinary BB-50 concentration was studied in 40 workers, with an average urine mercury concentration of 46 μg/g creatinine and who were exposed for an average of 7 years (Mutti et al., 1985), and 36 matched control workers. There was no difference between exposed and non-exposed workers in average urinary albumin or retinol-binding protein. However, when the 20 workers with urinary mercury above 50 μg/g creatinine were analysed separately, a shift of the BB-50 distribution towards higher values was found by a chi-square test (p = 0.07).

A study of 509 infants exposed to phenylmercury from contaminated diapers (Gotelli et al., 1985) showed a clear dose-response relationship between inorganic mercury in urine and urinary excretion of γ-glutamyl transpeptidase, an enzyme in the brush borders of the renal tubular cells.

Since phenylmercury compounds are known to be rapidly degraded to inorganic mercury in animals (Magos et al., 1982), it is likely that the renal effect in the infants was caused by inorganic mercury. Apart from the increased enzyme excretion, the children with the highest exposure also had increased 24-h urine volume. The enzyme excretion increased at a urine mercury excretion of 4 μg/kg body weight and the urine volume increased at 14 μg/kg body weight.

9.4 Skin reactions

9.4.1 Contact dermatitis

Primary hypersensitivity to metallic mercury is considered rare (Burrows, 1986). However, Thiomersal (sodium ethylmercurithiosalicilate) and ammoniated mercury have been found to be common sensitizers in a survey on the epidemiology of contact dermatitis (North American Contact Dermatitis Group, 1973), Thiomersal being the third commonest sensitizer (after nickel and chromium) in the general population. Both aryl- and alkylmercurial seed dressings have also been shown to be potent skin sensitizers. Mercury compounds give rise to a type IV cell-mediated delayed hypersensitivity reaction (Coombs & Gell, 1975).

There have been a few cases of allergic dermatitis among dental personnel (White & Brandt, 1976; Rudzki, 1979; Ancona et al., 1982). Patch testing of dental students (White & Brandt, 1976) indicated that the prevalence rate of mercury hypersensitivity increased by class from prefreshmen to seniors, successive values being 2.0%, 5.2%, 4.1%, 10.3%, and 10.8%. However, in a subsequent study (Miller et al., 1987), similar results were not found, but positive results from patch testing increased in relation to the number of amalgam restorations in the students. The overall percentage of positive reactions to mercuric chloride was very high (32%), which may indicate methodological problems. In this study, as in the study of White & Brandt (1976), the patch testing was carried out with 0.5 ml of a 0.1% aqueous solution of mercuric chloride.

Symptoms have occasionally been reported to relate to amalgam fillings (Frykholm, 1957; Thomson & Russell, 1970; Duxbury et al., 1982; SOS, 1987). In most cases the main

4

symptoms were facial dermatitis, sometimes with erythematous and urticarial rashes. Symptoms from the mouth (oral lichen planus) occasionally occurred. The symptoms started a few hours after the insertion of amalgam. Nakayama et al. (1983) reported 15 cases of generalized dermatitis caused by mercury after exposure from broken thermometers or dental treatment. In another very recent study employing epicutaneous testing, positive mercury hypersensitivity reactions were confined to subjects having preexisting amalgam restorations (Stenman & Bergman, 1989).

Finne et al. (1982) performed patch tests on 29 patients with amalgam fillings and oral lichen planus. Contact allergy was found in 62% of the subjects, compared with 3.2% in a control group. In four of the patients, all the amalgam restorations were removed and replaced by gold and composite materials. The lesions healed completely in three of these patients after an observation period of one year, and in the remaining case there was considerable improvement.

When peripheral blood lymphocytes from non-atopic subjects were cultured in the presence of pokeweed mitogen and mercuric chloride, a significant enhancement of the production of total IgE was observed, whereas the production of IgM and IgA remained unaffected (Kimata et al., 1983).

9.4.2 Pink disease and other skin manifestations

In the 1940s, "Pink disease" (acrodynia) was reported in children below 5 years of age as a result of the use of mercurous chloride in teething powder and ointments. Affected children became irritable and generally miserable and had difficulty in sleeping. Profuse sweating, photophobia, and generalized rash followed. The extremities became cold, painful, red, and swollen, and the skin desquamated. Neither the occurrence of this disease nor its severity was dose related. The urinary excretion of mercury in affected children was elevated but below the toxic level. After the withdrawal of teething powder preparations by the main United Kingdom manufacturers in 1953, there was a dramatic decline in the occurrence of Pink disease. Calomel is not the only mercurial that can cause Pink disease. Mercury dispersed from broken fluorescent bulbs (Tunnessen et al., 1987), long-term injection of γ-globulin preserved with ethylmercurithiosalicylate (Matheson et al., 1980), and the use of nappies treated with phenylmercury (Gotelli et al., 1985) have also been responsible for Pink disease. Exposure to mercury vapour may be associated with the mucocutaneous lymph node syndrome or "Kawasaki disease", which has many similarities with Pink disease (Orlowski & Mercer, 1980). Although the pathogenesis of Pink disease and Kawasaki disease is unknown, there is good evidence that Kawasaki disease is immunologically mediated, increased serum IgE concentrations and eosinophilia having been reported (Kusakawa & Heiner, 1976; Orlowski & Mercer, 1980; Adler et al., 1982). In Kawasaki disease, urinary mercury excretion is not always elevated, whereas it is in Pink disease.

9.5 Carcinogenicity

Inorganic mercury is generally not considered to be carcinogenic in humans (Kazantzis, 1981; Kazantzis & Lilly, 1986). However, recent observations have shown an excess risk of glioblastoma among Swedish dentists and dental nurses (Ahlbom et al., 1986). Based on the Swedish Cancer Environment Registry covering the years 1961-1979, a standardized morbidity ratio of 2.1 was observed (with 95% confidence limits 1.3-3.4). The authors concluded that the most probable origin is some occupational factor common to dentists and dental nurses, e.g., amalgam, chloroform, or radiography.

Cragle et al. (1984) published results of a mortality study of men exposed to elemental mercury. It was a retrospective cohort study of 5663 workers selected from about 14 000 workers in the Y-12 plant in Oak Ridge, USA, originally working on the Manhattan Project but later in a programme to produce large quantities of enriched lithium. Elemental mercury was used in the lithium isotope separation process. Mercury urinalysis testing started in mid-1953. Urine concentrations were not reported, but air mercury levels in 50-80% of the samples taken during the early 1950s were above 100 $\mu g/m^3$. The workers studied were divided into three groups: two exposed groups and one non-exposed group. It is not possible to evaluate the design as no valid exposure and selection data were presented. In all three groups, elevated SMRs (2.3, 1.2, 2.1) for tumours of the central nervous system were found. However, a statistically significant increase was reported only for the group consisting of 3260 non-mercury workers.

9.6 Mutagenicity and related end-points

WHO (1976) did not report any studies showing that inorganic mercury was genotoxic to humans. However, relevant data have since been reported. Popescu et al. (1979) compared four men exposed to elemental mercury vapour with a control group and found an increased prevalence of chromosomal aberrations. Verschaeve et al. (1976) and Verschaeve & Susanne (1979) showed an increase in aneuploidy after exposure to very low concentrations of metallic mercury vapour, but this could not be repeated in a later study (Verschaeve et al., 1979). Similarly, Mabille et al. (1984) did not find an increase of structural chromosomal aberrations in peripheral blood lymphocytes of workers exposed to metallic mercury vapour.

9.7 Dental amalgam and general health

During recent years there has been intense debate in some countries (e.g., Sweden and USA) on the possible health hazards of dental amalgams (Ziff, 1984; Penzer, 1986; SOS, 1987; Berglund, 1989). Those who claim that mercury from amalgam may cause severe health hazards refer to information on the release of mercury from amalgam and subsequent uptake into the body due to inhalation and swallowing of mercury. They also claim that a large number of people suffer from a variety of complaints and that their symptoms are caused by mercury. Those who deny a causal relation between dental amalgams and health effects point out that amalgam has been used for many years with no proven health effects. Furthermore, the uptake of mercury from amalgam is considerably less than has been associated with effects after occupational exposure to mercury (Fan, 1987).

There are many people with sometimes clearly incapacitating complaints who believe that these are caused by dental amalgam. Reports describing different types of symptoms or other effects (Hansson, 1986; Johansson & Lindh, 1987; Siblerud, 1988) do not allow any conclusions to be reached concerning their cause. This was also the opinion of a Swedish Task Group (SOS, 1987). The symptomatic picture is highly diverse and characterized by a variety of different symptoms. Some studies reported that patients improved after their amalgam fillings were replaced by another dental filling material. However, these reports have not been controlled for potential placebo effects.

Recently results from one epidemiological study have been reported by Ahlqwist et al. (1988). The data collection was carried out during 1980-1981. The majority of participants (85%) consisted of individuals who had already in 1968-69 participated in a longitudinal descriptive study of different diseases among women in the city of Gothenburg, Sweden. The remainder were included to expand the age strata and obtain a sample representative of women of the same age in the general population. Altogether 1024 women (aged 38-72 years) participated in the study, which covered a dental examination with an orthopantomogram and a medical examination including a standardized self-administered questionnaire regarding different symptoms or complaints. The dental and medical examinations were made by different people and without mentioning possible relations between amalgam and health risks. No positive correlations were found between number of amalgam fillings and number of symptoms or between number of amalgam fillings and prevalence of specified single symptoms or complaints. On the contrary, there were several age-matched significant correlations in the opposite direction. Some of these correlations (abdominal pain, poor appetite) disappeared when adjustment was made for number of teeth. Risk ratios (including 95% confidence limits) for women with 20 fillings or more compared to women with 0-4 fillings are given in Table 5. The authors concluded that their results do not support a correlation between number of surfaces with amalgam fillings and various symptoms studied on the population level. They do not exclude the possibility of a connection between amalgam fillings and special symptoms and complaints on the individual level, but, if such a connection exists, it has a low prevalence among the general population.

Table 5. Risk ratio for a specific symptom or complaint for 460 women
with 20 or more fillings compared to 193 women with 0-4 fillings[a]

Symptom or complaint	Risk ratio analysis	
	Risk ratio	95% confidence limits for risk ratio
Dizziness	0.70	0.46-1.07
Eye complaints	1.01	0.64-1.57
Hearing defects	0.66	0.41-1.07
Headache	1.22	0.83-1.80
General fatigue	0.79	0.55-1.15
Sleep disturbances	1.38	0.94-2.03
Nervous symptoms	0.80	0.52-1.25
Sweating	0.86	0.57-1.32
Breathlessness	0.65	0.41-1.03
Chest pain	0.62	0.39-0.99
Cough	0.71	0.47-1.08
Irritability	0.68	0.45-1.02
Over-exertion	0.60	0.38-0.96
Reduced mental concentration capacity	0.74	0.47-1.18
Restlessness	0.70	0.45-1.09
Depressive symptoms	0.74	0.50-1.07
Readiness to crying	0.72	0.46-1.11
Reduced ability to relax	1.15	0.79-1.69
Abdominal pain	0.64	0.42-0.98
Indisposition	1.00	0.57-1.76
Diarrhoea	0.62	0.32-1.18
Constipation	0.82	0.50-1.37
Poor appetite	0.33	0.16-0.68
Loss of weight	0.27	0.10-0.70
Overweight	0.76	0.52-1.12
Sensitivity to cold	0.78	0.50-1.21
Micturation disturbances	0.66	0.30-1.43
Joint complaints	0.97	0.66-1.43
Back complaints	0.74	0.51-1.07
Leg complaints	0.74	0.51-1.09

[a] The analysis was confined to dentulous women. Age was taken into consideration by means of the Mantel-Haenszel procedure. Modified from Ahlqwist et al. (1988).

Lavstedt & Sundberg (1989) investigated possible associations between dental amalgam and a range of symptoms by re-examining certain dental, medical, and sociological data originally collected from 1204 subjects in 1970 (i.e. prior to the present debate on dental amalgam). Standardization was made for various confounding factors, such as gender, social group, and smoking habits. There was no statistically significant increase in the percentage of individuals with symptoms in groups with increased numbers of amalgam fillings after controlling for confounding factors. The authors pointed out that the study did not exclude a causal association on the individual level. One strength of the study was that practically all of the examinations were carried out by one single investigator.

9.8 Reproduction, embryotoxicity, and teratogenicity

9.8.1 Occupational exposure

9.8.1.1 In males

McFarland & Reigel (1978) reported medical findings in nine men exposed accidentally for less than 8 h when more than 10 ml of mercury was instantly vapourized at a high temperature. Air mercury concentrations were estimated to be 44.3 mg/m^3. Even if these theoretical estimates are very uncertain, the exposure must have been extremely high. Six of the cases developed symptoms of acute poisoning. During a follow-up lasting several years they also showed signs of chronic poisoning. A loss of libido, which persisted for at least several years, was reported in all six cases.

Lauwerys et al. (1985) compared the fertility of 103 male workers, exposed to elemental mercury vapour in a zinc-mercury amalgam factory, a chloralkali plant, and in plants manufacturing electrical equipment, with 101 well-matched controls. The exposed group had an average blood mercury level of 14.6 μg/litre (SD 11.6 μg/litre) and an average urine mercury concentration of 52.4 μg/g creatinine (SD 46.7 μg/g). In the exposed group, 59 children were born compared to 65.8 expected (as calculated from data in the control group). However, the difference was not statistically significant.

In a study carried out at a US Department of Energy plant that used very large quantities of elemental mercury from 1953 to 1963, reproductive outcomes were studied among 247 male workers exposed to metallic mercury vapour (Alcser et al., 1989). As controls, 255 plant workers whose job did not require exposure to elemental mercury were used. No associations were demonstrated between mercury exposure and decreased fertility, increased rates of major malformations among the offspring, or serious childhood disease. There was an association between exposure and miscarriage, which disappeared however after controlling for the number of previous miscarriages before exposure began. The 95% adjusted confidence limits were 0.97–1.18. The authors pointed out certain problems with the study. The most serious methodological weakness in the evaluation was the necessity for subject recall of events that occurred 20 to 50 years previously. Another problem, which was not considered, was possible exposure to other toxic substances in the control group. The higher frequency of miscarriages among the exposed group prior to the exposure period could not be explained.

9.8.1.2 In females

There have been reports of increased menstrual disturbances in women exposed industrially or in dentistry to elemental mercury vapour. A study by De Rosis et al. (1985) examined a group of 106 women exposed to low levels of mercury (average values not exceeding 10 $\mu g/m^3$) and a control group of 241 unexposed women in another factory with similar working conditions. The percentage of women having normal menstrual cycles at the start of employment was very similar in both groups of women. During their period of employment more women in the exposed group noticed changes in the menstrual cycle than women in the control group. The age-standardized ratio of abnormal cycle frequency in exposed women to that in the control group was 1.4. The information was obtained by means of interviews, but these were not carried out on a blind basis. Therefore, according to the authors, the results neither prove nor exclude the possibility that occupational exposure to this concentration of mercury has a negative effect on the female reproductive system.

There have been reports which suggest that inorganic mercury compounds cause spontaneous abortion. Goncharuk (1977) reported that during a 4-year period 17% of 168 exposed workers in a mercury smelting plant had experienced spontaneous abortion (average exposure, 80 μg mercury per m^3), compared with 5% among 178 controls. Toxaemia during pregnancy was reported in 35% of the exposed and 2% of the unexposed workers. Gordon (1981) reported a slightly elevated incidence of spontaneous abortions among dentists. The results can not be interpreted with certainty, however, due to a non-response rate of almost 50%. The study of De Rosis et al. (1985), referred to earlier in this section, revealed no difference in the age-standardized rate of spontaneous abortion between mercury-exposed and unexposed female workers. Two other studies of female dental staff also reported no increased abortion rate when compared with age-standardized controls. In one of the studies (Heidam, 1984), the upper 95% confidence limit for odds ratio was about 2. In the other study (Brodsky et al., 1985), a comparison was made between a "low" exposure group and a "high" exposure group. The low exposure group comprised dental assistants preparing less than 40 amalgam restorations per week and the high exposure group those preparing more than 40 fillings a week. The assumed difference in exposure between the groups was not validated by measurements.

Two studies, one from Poland and one from Sweden, both dealing with spontaneous abortions and malformations, are of particular interest. The Polish study (Sikorski et al., 1987) revealed a high frequency of malformations among dental staff. Of 117 pregnancies in the mercury-exposed group, 28 pregnancies in 19 women led to reproductive failure, such as spontaneous abortion (19 cases, 16.2%), stillbirth (3 cases, 2.6%), congenital malformations (5 cases of spina bifida, 5.1%; one case of intra-atrial defect). This contrasts, in non-exposed controls, with seven cases of adverse pregnancy outcome (11.1%) in five women out of a total of 63 pregnancies (30 women). There were no malformations among the controls (R. Sikorski, personal communication to the IPCS). The age distribution of exposed and control women and the number of pregnancies before exposure or effect were not reported, which makes it difficult to interpret the data. For most countries the average rate of spina bifida is 5-10 (or less) per 10 000 births (International Clearing-house for Birth Defects Monitoring System, 1985) over a wide age span. Sikorski et al. (1987) reported a correlation between mercury levels in hair and reproductive failure in the exposed group. The meaning of this correlation is difficult to interpret, as hair is not a good indicator of exposure to metallic mercury vapour, due to several factors, including the possibility of external contamination (section 6.5.2). There is reason to believe, however, that the exposure was higher in the group with higher hair mercury levels (R. Sikorski, personal communication to the IPCS). Only 13.6% of the women studied used automatic amalgamators. The remaining 86.4% prepared the amalgam in an open mortar and almost never in separate rooms.

The Swedish study was reported by Ericson & Källén (1989), linking data from the Swedish National registers for birth records, malformations, and occupation. Altogether, 8157 children born to dentists (1360), dental nurses (6340), and dental technicians (457) were compared with the total number of births in Sweden during the observation period (1976, 1982-1986). The analysis took into consideration different confounding variables, such as the age of the mother and number of children. The study also examined the occurrence of stillbirths and spontaneous and induced abortions treated in hospitals. There was no tendency towards an elevated rate of malformation, abortion, or stillbirth. The study did not verify the high risk of spina bifida described in the Polish study (Sikorski et al., 1987). In spite of the large study group, the upper 95% confidence limit for the risk ratio of spina bifida was high (2.1), and the upper confidence limit of the absolute risk was about 1 per 1000 births. Therefore, the study is not a strong argument against an effect. In addition, a sample of 3991 pregnancies from the 1960s (among them there were 13 dentists, 65 dental assistants, and 6 dental technicians) was studied but no effects on spontaneous abortion rate or malformation was seen. The authors point out, however, that the only malformed infant observed had anencephaly and that both parents worked as dental technicians.

Among dental nurses, there was a significant excess of children with a birth weight of 2 to 2.5 kg. In total there were 274 children weighing less than 2.5 kg (against an expected number of 233), which gives a risk ratio for low birth weight of 1.2 (with a 95% confidence interval of 1.0-1.3). No similar excess in low birth weight was seen among dentists or dental technicians. Possible confounding socioeconomic factors, e.g., smoking, were not studied, but the authors suggested that these findings could be explained by differences in socioeconomic status.

During recent years much interest has focused on subclinical developmental changes in children exposed *in utero* or in early childhood to methylmercury and lead. No similar studies have been reported for inorganic mercury.

10. EVALUATION OF HUMAN HEALTH RISKS

Mercury exists in different forms, including elemental mercury, inorganic mercury and organic mercury compounds. They have some properties in common but differ in metabolism and toxicity. Biotransformation takes place in the body, particularly the transformation of metallic mercury vapour to mercuric compounds, which means that some of the effects of inorganic mercury could also be expected after exposure to metallic mercury vapour. There are, however, no empirical data showing whether or not inorganic mercury formed due to a biotransformation has similar toxicity and metabolism to that of inorganic mercury accumulated in the body as a result of exposure to inorganic mercury itself. It would be prudent to consider, until more information is available, that, with the exception of acute renal tubular cell damage, the two forms of inorganic mercury have similar toxicity.

10.1 Exposure levels and routes

10.1.1 Mercury vapour

Human long-term exposure to mercury vapour is primarily encountered in an occupational setting and in cases where the metal has been handled inappropriately in the home. Continual low-level exposure to mercury vapour occurs in the mouth in the presence of dental amalgam fillings. The amount of mercury vapour released intra-orally depends on the number, surface area, and mechanical loading of the amalgam restorations. Atmospheric levels of mercury found in the workplace, e.g., chloralkali plants, are usually below 50 $\mu g/m^3$. Levels above 50 $\mu g/m^3$ and even exceeding 100 $\mu g/m^3$ can be found in work environments where good industrial hygiene has not been practiced or in home operations, in which the highest levels would be expected. Values for air concentration (in $\mu g/m^3$) are approximately the same as those for urine mercury concentration (expressed in $\mu g/g$ creatinine). The use of urinary mercury excretion makes it possible to compare intake from the working atmosphere and release from dental amalgam.

Occupational exposure to mercury vapour in dentistry has been well established, reported exposure levels being

4-30 $\mu g/m^3$, on average, with up to 150-170 $\mu g/m^3$ in some clinics. The values for mean intraoral mercury vapour concentration derived from dental amalgam have been reported to be in the range of 3 to 29 $\mu g/m^3$.

Approximately 80% of inhaled mercury vapour is absorbed from the lungs, while uptake of mercury vapour via the skin is about 1% of uptake by inhalation. No data are available on the possible oral mucosal absorption of mercury vapour. Mercury vapour can cross the plancental barrier, thus exposing the developing fetus.

10.1.2 Inorganic mercury compounds

The major source of high exposure to humans from mercuric compounds involves medicaments, both traditional and alternative, and skin-lightening creams and soaps. There is some evidence from occupational settings where chlorine is used that a part of the mercury vapour can be transformed in the atmosphere and absorbed as an aerosol of mercuric mercury. Mercuric mercury is to a great extent deposited in the placenta, where it causes damage that may lead to adverse effects on the fetus.

Mercurous mercury, in the form of calomel, has for long been used in therapeutics. The mercury content in the brain of two daily users of calomel, ingesting 240 mg mercurous chloride per day, was 4-106 mg/kg brain, indicating that elemental mercury is formed from mercurous chloride following ingestion.

10.2 Toxic effects

10.2.1 Mercury vapour

Over-exposure to mercury vapour gives rise to neurological effects with initially a fine high-frequency intention tremor and neurobehavioural impairment. Peripheral nerve involvement has also been observed. Proteinuria and lysosomal enzymes in the urine of exposed workers indicate an effect on the kidney of chloralkali workers; the presence of mercuric mercury may have contributed to this effect. The nephrotic syndrome has been reported among chloralkali workers. Pink disease, skin allergy, and mucocutaneous lymph node syndrome (Kawasaki disease) in children, have also been observed after exposure to mercury vapour.

Hypersensitivity skin reactions have been described after exposure to metallic mercury vapour from mercury amalgam materials. No data supporting carcinogenic effects of mercury vapour have been reported. There has been a report of excess risk of glioblastoma observed in Swedish dental personnel. At this stage, however, it has not been possible to associate this excess risk with any specific group of dental materials. The standard of published epidemiological studies is such that it remains an open question whether mercury vapour can adversely affect the menstrual cycle or fetal development in the absence of the well-known signs of mercury intoxication.

10.2.2 *Inorganic mercury compounds*

Information on pulmonary deposition and absorption of mercuric mercury aerosols is lacking. However, it is likely that significant absorption takes place directly from the lung and probably from the gastrointestinal tract after mucociliary clearance from the lung.

Most adverse effects of mercuric compounds in humans have been reported after oral ingestion or skin absorption. However, only limited information is available as far as dose-effect relationships are concerned. From animal experiments it is possible to identify the critical lowest effect levels that are likely to result in proteinuria in humans after chronic exposure. Proteinuria in humans is believed to be produced through the formation of mercuric-mercury-induced autoimmune glomerulonephritis. The production and deposition of IgG antibodies to glomerular basement membrane can be considered the first step in the formation of this glomerulonephritis. No data on possible carcinogenic effects of mercuric mercury have been reported.

10.3 Dose-response relationships

10.3.1 *Mercury vapour*

The risk assessment of exposure to mercury vapour is hindered by the heterogeneity of published data, problems with the estimation of exposure (e.g., lack of speciation and methodological uncertainties), uncertainty concerning the reliability of subjective symptoms, and the selection of control groups for comparison with low exposure groups.

Nevertheless the data presented in section 9 allow a broad characterization to be made.

a) When exposure is above 80 $\mu g/m^3$, corresponding to a urine mercury level of 100 $\mu g/g$ creatinine (section 6.5.2), the probability of developing the classical neurological signs of mercury intoxication (tremor, erethism) and proteinuria is high.

b) Exposure in the range of 25 to 80 $\mu g/m^3$, corresponding to a level of 30 to 100 μg mercury/g creatinine, increases the incidence of certain less severe toxic effects that do not lead to overt clinical impairment. These subtle effects are defects in psychomotor performance, objectively detectable tremor, and evidence of impaired nerve conduction velocity, which are present only in particularly sensitive individuals. The occurrence of several subjective symptoms, such as fatigue, irritability, and loss of appetite, is also increased. In a few studies, tremor, recorded electrophysiologically, has been observed at low urine concentrations (down to 25-35 $\mu g/g$ creatinine). Other studies did not show such an effect. Although the incidence of some signs was increased in this exposure range, most studies did not find a dose-response relationship. Some of the exposed people develop proteinuria (proteins of low relative molecular mass and microalbuminuria). The available studies are generally of small size and low statistical power.

c) Appropriate epidemiological data covering exposure levels corresponding to less than 30-50 μg mercury per g creatinine are not available. Since a specific no-observed-effect level cannot be established and if larger populations are exposed to low concentrations of mercury, it cannot be excluded that mild adverse effects may occur in certain sensitive individuals.

Some studies have found miscarriages and abortions after occupational exposure to mercury, but other studies did not confirm these effects. The WHO Study Group in 1980 stated: "The exposure of women of child-bearing age to mercury vapour should be as low as possible. The Group was not in a position to recommend a specific value" (WHO, 1980). This statement is still prudent and will remain so until new data become available.

10.3.2 Inorganic mercury compounds

The risk assessment of exposure to inorganic mercury compounds is hindered by a lack of adequate human data dealing with the relationship between dose and effects/ responses. For this reason, more human research is needed in order to arrive at the goal of a human risk evaluation of inorganic mercuric mercury compounds at low levels.

The intake of gram doses of mercuric chloride causes severe to lethal renal tubular damage and necrosis of the gastrointestinal mucous membrane. At lower dose levels, less pronounced tubular damage occurs, reflected in amino-aciduria, increased diuresis, and loss of renal enzymes in the urine.

A special problem in the risk assessment of mercury is the fact that mercury can give rise to allergic and immunotoxic reactions, which are partly genetically regulated. There may well be a small fraction of the population that is particularly sensitive, as has been observed in animal studies. A consequence of an immunological etiology is that it is not scientifically possible to set a level for mercury, e.g., in blood or urine, below which mercury-related symptoms will not occur in individual cases, since dose-response studies for groups of immunologically sensitive individuals are not yet available.

Based upon the evaluation in animals, the most sensitive adverse effect for inorganic mercury risk assessment is the formation of mercuric-mercury-induced auto-immune glomerulonephritis, the first step being the production and deposition of IgG antibodies to the glomerular basement membrane. The Brown Norway rat is a good test species for the study of mercuric-mercury-induced auto-immune glomerulonephritis (although this effect has also been observed in rabbits), and it is the best animal model for the study of mercury-induced kidney damage at present. The group of studies presented in Table 4 (section 8.2.2.6) was selected for consideration of mercuric mercury risk assessment. A no-observed-adverse-effect level (NOAEL) could not be determined from these animal studies. The lowest-observed-adverse-effect level (LOAEL) was found in the subcutaneous exposure study by Druet et al. (1978). In this study, subcutaneous doses of mercuric chloride (0.05 mg/kg body weight three times per week) were administered for 12 weeks and resulted in antibodies being bound to the glomerular basement membrane of the rat kidney.

Using this animal LOAEL (0.05 mg/kg), equivalent human oral and inhalation LOAEL values for kidney effects can be determined as follows:

Average daily subcutaneous dose:

$$= \frac{(0.05 \text{ mg/kg}) \times 3 \text{ days} \times 0.739}{7 \text{ days}} = 0.0158 \text{ mg/kg per day}$$

where: 0.05 mg/kg = dose of $HgCl_2$ injected subcutaneously into rats
3 days = number of days per week that doses were administered
7 days = number of days per week
0.739 = fraction of $HgCl_2$ that is Hg^{2+} ion.

Although the calculated values have been rounded, the un-rounded values were always used in subsequent calculations.

Human oral exposure equivalent determination:

$$= \frac{(0.0158 \text{ mg/kg per day}) \times 70 \text{ kg} \times 100\%}{7\%} = 15.8 \text{ mg/day}$$

where: 0.0158 mg/kg per day = average daily subcutaneous dose of Hg^{2+}
70 kg = assumed body weight of an adult human
100% = assumed percentage of Hg^{2+} absorbed from the subcutaneous route of exposure
7% = assumed percentage of Hg^{2+} absorbed from the oral route of exposure

Human inhalation exposure equivalent determination:

a) For 24-h general population exposure:

$$\frac{(0.0158 \text{ mg/kg per day}) \times 70 \text{ kg} \times 100\%}{(20 \text{ m}^3/\text{day}) \times 80\%} = 0.069 \text{ mg/m}^3$$

where: 0.0158 mg/kg per day = average daily subcutaneous dose of Hg^{2+}
70 kg = assumed body weight of an adult
20 m^3/day = assumed volume of air inhaled during a 24-h period
100% = assumed percentage of Hg^{2+} absorbed from subcutaneous route of exposure
80% = assumed percentage of Hg^0 absorbed from the lung.

b) For 8-h work-day exposure:

$$\frac{(0.0158 \text{ mg/kg per day}) \times 70 \text{ kg} \times 100\%}{(10 \text{ m}^3/\text{day}) \times 80\%} = 0.139 \text{ mg/m}^3$$

where: 0.0158 mg/kg per day = average daily subcutaneous dose of Hg^{2+}
70 kg = assumed body weight of an adult
10 m^3 = assumed volume of air inhaled during a work-day
100% = assumed percentage of Hg^{2+} absorbed from subcutaneous route of exposure
80% = assumed percentage of Hg^0 absorbed from the lung.

These inhalation LOAEL values calculated for kidney effects are well within the range of mercury vapour exposures in humans where neurological and renal effects have been observed.

11. RECOMMENDATIONS FOR FURTHER RESEARCH

Further research is required in the following areas:

1. Determination of the exposure to different chemical forms of mercury at low levels of exposure, including the development of microtechniques for speciation of small quantities of mercury in biological materials and of analytical quality assurance techniques.

2. The pharmacokinetics of mercury release from amalgam restorations in relation to time, diet, technical and physiological conditions, and the development of tests for identifying specially sensitive individuals (e.g., local mucosa reactions, intra-oral electrochemical measurements, immunotoxicity).

3. The use of mercury compounds in pharmaceuticals and cosmetics.

4. The binding, biotransformation, and transport of different forms of mercury, both in animals and humans, including interactions with selenium.

5. The transplacental transport of mercury and specific distribution in fetal organs, fetotoxic effects, and developmental effects with emphasis on neurobehavioural effects.

6. Research on the neurobehavioural effects of mercury in the occupationally exposed population (dentists, etc.).

7. The epidemiology of the role of mercury in inducing glomerulonephritis in the general population.

8. The prevalence of immunological effects and hypersensitivity in low-dose exposure to mercury with or without subjective symptoms.

9. A case-control study of brain tumours, in particular glioblastoma, and exposure to mercury.

Measures to decrease the exposure of the general population to mercury-containing pharmaceuticals and cosmetics should be promoted.

12. PREVIOUS EVALUATIONS BY INTERNATIONAL BODIES

The human health risks of inorganic mercury compounds were previously evaluated in Environmental Health Criteria 1: Mercury (WHO, 1976). More recent evaluations by the International Programme on Chemical Safety (IPCS) have dealt mainly with the health risks of methylmercury exposure (WHO, 1990). A WHO review of the occupational health risks of inorganic mercury (WHO, 1980) and an IPCS review of the environmental aspects of mercury (WHO, 1989) have been published. The recommended health-based occupational exposure limit for metallic mercury vapour (WHO, 1980) is 25 μg mercury/m^3 air (TWA, long-term exposure) and 500 μg mercury/m^3 air (peaks, short-term exposure). The equivalent value for long-term exposure to inorganic mercury compounds is 50 μg mercury/m^3 air (TWA) (WHO, 1980). A maximum individual urine mercury concentration of 50 μg/g creatinine has also been recommended (WHO, 1980).

Regulatory standards established by national bodies in various countries and in the European Community are summarized in the data profile of the International Register of Potentially Toxic Chemicals (IRPTC, 1987).

REFERENCES

ABRAHAM, J.E., SVARE, C.W., & FRANK, C.W. (1984) The effect of dental amalgam restorations on blood mercury levels. J. dent. Res., **63**(1): 71-73.

ADA (1985) Dental amalgam, Chicago, American Dental Association.

ADLER, R., BOXSTEIN, D., SCHAFF, P., & KELLY, D. (1982) Metallic mercury vapour poisoning stimulating mucocutaneous lymph node syndrome. J. Pediatr., **101**(6): 967-968.

AGNER, E. & JANS, H. (1978) Mercury poisoning and nephrotic syndrome in two young siblings. Lancet, **II**: 951.

AGOCS, M.M., ETZEL, R.A., PARRISH, R.G., PASCHAL, D.C., CAMPAGNA, P.R., COHEN, D.S., KILBOURNE, E.M., & HESSE, J.L. (in press) Mercury exposure from interior latex paint. N. Engl. J. Med.

AHLBOM, A., NORELL, S., NYLANDER, M., & RODVALL, Y. (1986) Dentists, dental nurses, and brain tumours. Br. med. J., **292**: 662.

AHLQWIST, M., BENGTSSON, C., FURUNES, B., HOLLENDER, L., & LAPIDUS, L. (1988) Number of amalgam tooth fillings in relation to subjectively experienced symptoms in a study of Swedish women. Community dent. oral Epidemiol., **16**: 227-231.

AITIO, A. (1988) Biological monitoring. In: Clarkson, T., Friberg, L., Nordberg, G., & Sager, P., ed. Biological monitoring of toxic metals, New York, London, Plenum Press, pp. 75-83.

AITIO, A., VALKONEN, S., KIVISTÖ, H., & YRJÄNHEIKKI, E. (1983) Effect of occupational mercury exposure on plasma lysosomal hydrolases. Int. Arch. occup. environ. Health, **53**: 139-147.

ALBERS, J.W., KALLENBACH, L.R., FINE, L.J., LANGOLF, G.D., WOLFE, R.A., DONOFRIO, P.D., ALESSI, A.G., STOLP-SMITH, K.A., BROMBERG, M.B., & THE MERCURY WORKERS STUDY GROUP (1988) Neurological abnormalities associated with remote occupational elemental mercury exposure. Ann. Neurol., **24**: 651-659.

ALCSER, K.H., BRIX, K.A., FINE, L.J., KALLENBACH, L.R., & WOLFE, R.A. (1989) Occupational mercury exposure and male reproductive health. Am. J. Ind. Med., **15**(5): 517-529.

ALEXANDER, J., THOMASSEN, Y., & AASETH, J. (1983) Increased urinary excretion of selenium among workers exposed to elemental mercury vapor. J. appl. Toxicol., **3**(3): 143-145.

ANCONA, A., RAMOS, M., SUAREZ, R., & MACOTELA, E. (1982) Mercury sensitivity in a dentist. Contact dermatitis, **8**: 218.

ANDERSEN, O., RONNE, M., & NORDBERG, G.F. (1983) Effects of inorganic metal salts on chromosome length in human lymphocytes. Hereditas, **98**: 65-70.

ANDRES, P. (1984) IgA-IgG disease in the intestine of Brown-Norway rats ingesting mercuric chloride. Clin. Immunol. Immunopathol., 30: 488-494.

AOI, T., HIGUCHI, T., KIDOKORO, R., FUKUMURA, R., YAGI, A., OHGUCHI, S., SASA, A., HAYASHI, H., SAKAMOTO, N., & HANAICHI, T. (1985) An association of mercury with selenium in inorganic mercury intoxication. Hum. Toxicol., 4: 637-642.

ARONSSON, M.A., LIND, B., NYLANDER, M., & NORDBERG, M. (1989) Dental amalgam and mercury. Biol. Metals, 2: 25-30.

ARVIDSON, B. (1987) Research note. Retrograde axonal transport of mercury. Exper. Neurol., 98: 198-203.

ASHE, W., LARGENT, E., DUTRA, F., HUBBARD, D., & BLACKSTONE, M. (1953) Behaviour of mercury in the animal organism following inhalation. Ind. med. occup. Med., 22: 19-43.

ATSDR (1989) Toxicological profile for mercury. Atlanta, Agency for Toxic Substances and Disease Registry (US Public Health Service).

ATEN, J., BOSMAN, C.B., ROZING, J., STIJNEN, T., HOEDEMAEKER, Ph.J., & WEENING, J.J. (1988) Mercuric chloride-induced autoimmunity in the Brown Norway rat: cellular kinetics and major histocompatibility complex antigen expression. Am. J. Pathol., 133(1): 127-138.

BARIETY, J., DRUET, P., LALIBERTE, F., & SAPIN, C. (1971) Glomerulonephritis with gamma- and beta1C-globulin deposits induced in rats by mercuric chloride. Am. J. Pathol., 65: 293-302.

BARNES, J.L., MCDOWELL, E.M., MCNEIL, J.S., FLAMENBAUM, W., & TRUMP, B.F. (1980) Studies on the pathophysiology of acute renal failure. IV. Protective effect of dithiothreitol following administration of mercuric chloride in the rat. Virchows Arch. cell Pathol., 32: 201-232.

BARR, R.D., REES, P.H., CORDY, P.E., KUNGU, A., WOODGER, B.A., & CAMERON, H.M. (1972) Nephrotic syndrome in adult Africans in Nairobi. Br. med. J., 2: 131-134.

BARR, R.D., WOODGER, B.A., & REES, P.H. (1973) Levels of mercury in urine correlated with the use of skin lightening creams. Am. J. clin. Pathol., 59: 36-40.

BATTISTONE, G.C., HEFFERREN, J.J., MILLER, R.A., & CUTRIGHT, D.E. (1976) Mercury: its relation to the dentist's health and dental practice characteristics. J. Am. Dent. Assoc., 92: 1182-1188.

BAUER, J.G. & FIRST, H.A. (1982) The toxicity of mercury in dental amalgam. California dent. J., 47-61.

BELLON, B., CAPRON, M., DRUET, E., VERROUST, P., VIAL, M.C., SAPIN, C., GIRARD, J.F., FOIDART, J.M., MAHIEU, P., & DRUET, P. (1982) Mercuric chloride induced autoimmune disease in Brown-Norway rats:

Sequential search for anti-basement membrane antibodies and circulating immune complexes. Eur. J. clin. Invest., **12**: 127-133.

BERGLUND, A., POHL, L., OLSSON, S., & BERGMAN, M. (1988) Determination of the rate of release of intra-oral mercury vapor from amalgam. J. dent. Res., **67**(9): 1235-1242.

BERGLUND, F. (1989) [Amalgam poisoning, a medical reality.] Läkartidningen, **86**(1-2): 41-42 (in Swedish).

BERLIN, M. & JOHANSSON, L.G. (1964) Mercury in mouse brain after inhalation of mercury vapour and after intravenous injection of mercury salts. Nature, London, **204**: 85-86.

BERLIN, M., FAZACKERLEY, J., & NORDBERG, G. (1969) The uptake of mercury in the brains of mammals exposed to mercury vapor and mercuric salts. Arch. environ. Health, **18**: 719-729.

BERLIN, M., CARLSON, J., & NORSETH, T. (1975) Dose-dependence of methyl-mercury metabolism. A study of distribution: biotransformation and excretion in the Squirrel Monkey. Arch. environ. Health, **30**: 307-313.

BERNARD, A.M., ROELS, H.R., FOIDART, J.M., & LAUWERYS, R.L. (1987) Search for anti-laminin antibodies in the serum of workers exposed to cadmium, mercury vapour or lead. Int. Arch. occup. environ. Health, **59**: 303-309.

BERNARD, S.R. & PURDUE, P. (1984) Metabolic models for methyl and inorganic mercury. Health Phys., **46**(3): 695-699.

BERNAUDIN, J.F., DRUET, E., DRUET, P., & MASSE, R. (1981) Inhalation or ingestion of organic or inorganic mercurials produces auto-immune disease in rats. Clin. Immunol. Immunopathol., **20**: 129-135.

BIDSTRUP, P.L., BONNEL, J.A., HARVEY, D.G., & LOCKET, S. (1951) Chronic mercury poisoning in men repairing direct-current meters. Lancet, **2**: 856-861.

BONDY, S.C., ANDERSON, C.L., HARRINGTON, M.E., & PRASAD, K.N. (1979) The effects of organic and inorganic lead and mercury on neurotrans-mitter high-affinity transport and release mechanisms. Environ. Res., **19**: 102-111.

BOWMAN, C., MASON, D.W., PUSEY, C.D., & LOCKWOOD, C.M. (1984) Auto-regulation of autoantibody synthesis in mercuric chloride nephritis in the Brown-Norway rat. I. A role for T suppressor cells. Eur. J. Immunol., **14**: 464-470.

BRADY, J.A., GEMMITI-NUNN, D., POLAN, A.K., MITCHELL, D., WEIL, R., & VIANNA, N.J. (1980) The relationship of dental practice characteristics to blood mercury levels. NY State dent. J., **46**: 420-424.

BRIGATTI, L. (1949) [Mercury levels in human organs with and without mercury exposure.] Med. Lav., **40**(10): 233-239 (in Italian).

BRODSKY, J.B., COHEN, E.N., WHITCHER, C., BROWN, B.W., Jr, & WU, M.L. (1985) Occupational exposure to mercury in dentistry and pregnancy outcome. J. Am. Dent. Assoc., 111: 779-780.

BRUNE, D. (1981) Corrosion of amalgams. Scand. J. dent. Res., 89: 506-514.

BRUNE, D. & EVJE, D.M. (1985) Man's mercury loading from a dental amalgam. Sci. total Environ., 44: 51-63.

BUCHET, J.P., ROELS, H., BERNARD, A., Jr, & LAUWERYS, R. (1980) Assessment of renal function of workers exposed to inorganic lead, cadmium or mercury vapor. J. occup. Med., 22(11): 741-750.

BUCHWALD, H. (1972) Exposure of dental workers to mercury. Am. Ind. Hyg. Assoc. J., 33: 492-502.

BUNN, W.B., MCGILL, C.M., BARBER, T.E., CROMER, J.W., Jr, & GOLDWATER, L.J. (1986) Mercury exposure in chloralkali plants. Am. Ind. Hyg. Assoc. J., 47(5): 249-254.

BURK, R.F., FOSTER, K.A., GREENFIELD, P.M., & KIKER, K.W. (1974) Binding of simultaneously administered inorganic selenium and mercury to a rat plasma protein (37894). Proc. Soc. Exp. Biol. Med., 145: 782-785.

BURROWS, D. (1986) Hypersensitivity to mercury, nickel and chromium in relation to dental materials. Int. dent. J., 36: 30-34.

CANTONI, O. & COSTA, M. (1983) Correlations of DNA strand breaks and their repair with cell survival following acute exposure to mercury (II) and X-rays. Mol. Pharmacol. 24: 84-89.

CANTONI, O., EVANS, R.M., & COSTA, M. (1982) Similarity in the acute cytotoxic response of mammalian cells to mercury (II) and X-rays: DNA damage and glutathione depletion. Biochem. Bioophys. Res. Commun., 108(2): 614-619.

CANTONI, O., CHRISTIE, N.T., ROBISON, S.H., & COSTA, M. (1984a) Characterization of DNA lesions produced by $HgCl_2$ in cell culture systems. Chem.-biol. Interact., 49: 209-224.

CANTONI, O., CHRISTIE, N.T., SWANN, A., DRATH, D.B., COSTA, M. (1984b) Mechanism of $HgCl_2$ cytotoxicity in cultured mammalian cells. Mol. Pharmacol., 26: 360-368.

CASSANO, G.B., AMADUCCI, L., & VIOLA, P.L. (1966) Distribution of mercury (H^{203}) in the brain of chronically intoxicated mice (autoradiographic study). Riv. Pat. nerv. ment., 87: 214-225.

CENTERS FOR DISEASE CONTROL (1990) Mercury exposure from interior latex paint. CDC Mortal. Morb. Wkly Rep., 39(8): 125-126.

CHALOPING, J.M. & LOCKWOOD, C.M. (1984) Autoregulation of auto-antibody synthesis in mercuric chloride nephritis in the Brown Norway rat. II. Presence of antigen-augmentable plaque-forming cells in the spleen is associated with humoral factors behaving as auto-anti-idiotypic antibodies. Eur. J. Immunol., **14**: 470-475.

CHANG, S.B., SIEW, C., & GRUNINGER, S.E. (1987) Examination of blood levels of mercurials in practicing dentists using cold-vapor atomic absorption spectrometry. J. anal. Toxicol., **11**: 149-153.

CHEN, R.W., WHANGER, P.D., & FANG, S.C. (1974) Diversion of mercury binding in rat tissues by selenium: A possible mechanism of protection. Pharmacol. Res. Commun., **6**(6): 571-579.

CHERIAN, M.G., HURSH, J.B., CLARKSON, T.W., & ALLEN, J. (1978) Radioactive mercury distribution in biological fluids and excretion in human subjects after inhalation of mercury vapor. Arch. environ. Health, **33**: 109-114.

CHMIELNICKA, J., BRZEZNICKA, E., & SNIADY, A. (1986) Kidney concentrations and urinary excretion of mercury, zinc and copper following the administration of mercuric chloride and sodium selenite to rats. Arch. Toxicol., **59**: 16-20.

CHOWDHURY, A.R., VACHHRAJANI, K.D., MAKHIJA, S., & KASHYAP, S.K. (1986) Histomorphometric and biochemical changes in the testicular tissues of rats treated with mercuric chloride. Biomed. Biochim. Acta, **45**(7): 949-956.

CHRISTIE, N.T., CANTONI, O., EVANS, R.M., MEYN, R.E., & COSTA, M. (1984) Use of mammalian DNA repair-deficient mutants to assess the effects of toxic metal compounds on DNA. Biochem. Pharmacol., **33**(10): 1661-1670.

CHRISTIE, N.T., CANTONI, O., SUGIYAMA, M., CATTEBENI, F., & COSTA, M. (1986) Differences in the effects of Hg(II) on DNA repair induced in Chinese hamster ovary cells by ultraviolet or X-rays. Mol. Pharmacol., **29**: 173-178.

CLARKSON, T.W. & KILPPER, R.W. (1978) The metabolism of inhaled vapor in animals and man. In: Clarkson, T.W., ed. Heavy metals as environmental hazards to man, Rochester, New York, Environmental Health Sciences Center Program Project, pp. 449A, 449B.

CLARKSON, T.W., MAGOS, L., & GREENWOOD, M.R. (1972) The transport of elemental mercury into fetal tissues. Biol. Neonate, **21**: 239-244.

CLARKSON, T.W., FRIBERG, L., HURSH, J.B., & NYLANDER, M. (1988a) The prediction of intake of mercury vapor from amalgams. In: Clarkson, T.W., Friberg, L., Nordberg, G.F., & Sager, P., ed. Biological monitoring of metals, New York, London, Plenum Press, pp. 247-264.

CLARKSON, T.W., HURSH, J.B., SAGER, P.R., & SYVERSEN, T.L.M. (1988b) Mercury. In: Clarkson, T.W., Friberg, L., Nordberg, G.F., & Sager, P., ed. Biological monitoring of metals, New York, London, Plenum Press, pp. 199-246.

CLARKSON, T.W., FRIBERG. L., NORDBERG., G.F., & SAGER, P. ed. (1988c) Biological monitoring of metals, New York, London, Plenum Press, 686 pp.

CLOEZ, I., DUMONT, O., PICIOTTI, M., & BOURRE, J.M. (1987) Alterations of lipid synthesis in the normal and dysmyelinating trembler mouse sciatic nerve by heavy metals (Hg, Pb, Mn, Cu, Ni). Toxicology, 46: 65-71.

COOLEY, R.L. & BARKMEIER, W.W. (1978) Mercury vapor emitted during ultraspeed cutting of amalgam. J. Indiana Dent. State Assoc., 57(2): 28-31.

COOMBS, R.R.A. & GELL, P.G.H. (1975) Classification of allergic reactions responsible for clinical hypersensitivity and disease. In: Gell, P.G.H., Coombs, R.R.A., & Lachmann, P.J. ed. Clinical aspects of immunology, 3rd ed., Oxford, London, Blackwell Scientific Publications, pp. 761-781.

COYLE, P. & HARTELY, T. (1981) Automated determination of mercury in urine and blood by the Magos reagent and cold vapor atomic absorption spectrometry. Anal. Chem., 53: 354-356.

CRAGLE, D.L., HOLLIS, D.R., QUALTERS, J.R., TANKERSLEY, W.G., & FRY, S.A. (1984) A mortality study of men exposed to elemental mercury. J. occup. Med., 26(11): 817-821.

CRC (1972) Handbook of chemistry and physics, 32nd ed., Cleveland, Ohio, CRC Press.

CROSS, J.D., DALE, I.M., GOOLVARD, L., LENIHAN, J.M.A., & SMITH, H. (1978) Methyl mercury in blood of dentists. Lancet, II: 312-313.

DASTON, G.P., KAVLOCK, R.J., ROGERS, E.H., & CARVER, B. (1983) Toxicity of mercuric chloride to the developing rat kidney. I. Postnatal ontogeny of renal sensitivity. Toxicol. appl. Pharmacol., 71: 24-41.

DAVIS, L.E., WANDS, J.R., WEISS, S.A., PRICE, D.L., & GIRLING, E.F. (1974) Central nervous system intoxication from mercurous chloride laxatives. Quantitative, histochemical and ultrastructural studies. Arch. Neurol., 30: 428-431.

DEAN, R.B. & SUESS, M.J. (1985) The risk to health of chemicals in sewage sludge applied to land. Waste Manage. and Res., 3: 251-278.

DE ROSIS, F., ANASTASIO, S.P., SELVAGGI, L., BELTRAME, A., & MORIANI, G. (1985) Female reproductive health in two lamp factories: Effects of exposure to inorganic mercury vapour and stress factors. Br. J. ind. Med., 42: 488-494.

DIAMOND, G.L. (1988) Biological monitoring of urine for exposure to toxic metals. In: Clarkson, T.W., Friberg, L., Nordberg, G.F., & Sager, P., ed. Biological monitoring of metals, New York, London, Plenum Press, pp. 515-529.

DRUET, E., SAPIN, C., GÜNTHER, E., FEINGOLD, N., & DRUET, P. (1977) Mercuric chloride-induced anti-glomerular basement membrane antibodies in the rat. Eur. J. Immunol., 7: 348-351.

DRUET, E., SAPIN, C., FOURNIE, G., MANDET, C., GUNTHER, E., & DRUET, P. (1982) Genetic control of susceptibility to mercury-induced immune nephritis in various strains of rat. Clin. Immunol. Immunopathol., **25**: 203-212.

DRUET, P., DRUET, E., POTDEVIN, F., & SAPIN, C. (1978) Immune type glomerulonephritis induced by $HgCl_2$ in the Brown Norway rat. Ann. Immunol., **129C**: 777-792.

DRUET, P., TEYCHENNE, P., MANDET, C., BASCOU, C., & DRUET, E. (1981) Immune-type glomerulonephritis induced in the Brown-Norway rat with mercury-containing pharmaceutical products. Nephron, **28**: 145-148.

DUMAREY, R., DAMS, R., & HOSTE, J. (1985) Comparison of the collection and desorption efficiency of activated charcoal, silver, and gold for the determination of vapor-phase atmospheric mercury. Anal. Chem., **57**(13): 2638-2643.

DUNN, J.D., CLARKSON, T.W., & MAGOS, L. (1978) Ethanol-increased exhalation of mercury in mice. Br. J. ind. Med., **35**: 241-244.

DUNN, J.D., CLARKSON, T.W., & MAGOS, L. (1981a) Ethanol reveals novel mercury detoxification step in tissues. Science, **213**: 1123-1125.

DUNN, J.D., CLARKSON, T.W., & MAGOS, L. (1981b) Interaction of ethanol and inorganic mercury: Generation of mercury vapor in vivo. J. Pharmacol. exp. Ther., **216**(1): 19-23.

DUXBURY, A.J., EAD, R.D., MCMURROUGH, S., & WATTS, D.C. (1982) Allergy to mercury in dental amalgam. Br. dent. J., **152**: 47-48.

EDIMED (1989) [The pharmaceutical informer. Italian directory of drugs and manufacturers], 50th ed., Milano, Organizzazione Editoriale Medico Farmaceutica (in Italian).

EGGLESTON, D.W. & NYLANDER, M. (1987) Correlation of dental amalgam with mercury in brain tissue. J. prosthet. Dent., **58**(6): 704-707.

EHRENBERG, R.L., BLAIR SMITH, A., MCMANUS, K.P., HANNON, W.H., BRIGHTWELL, W.S., LOWRY, L.K., ANGER, W.K., VOGT, R.L., BRONDUM, J., & HUDSON, P.J. (1986) Health hazard evaluation report, Cincinnati, Ohio, National Institute for Occupational Safety and Health, 65 pp. (HETA, 83-465-1674).

EICHHORN, G.L. & CLARK, P. (1963) The reaction of mercury (II) with nucleosides. J. Am. Chem. Soc., **85**: 4020-4024.

ELINDER, G.-G., GERHARDSSON, L., & OBERDOERSTER, G. (1988) Biological monitoring of metals. In: Clarkson, T.W., Friberg, L., Nordberg, G.F., & Sager, P., ed. Biological monitoring of metals, New York, London, Plenum Press, pp. 1-71.

ENWONWU, C.O. (1987) Potential health hazard of use of mercury in dentistry: Critical review of the literature. Environ. Res., **42**: 251-274.

ERICSON, A. & KÄLLÉN, B. (1988) Pregnancy outcome in women working as dentists, dental assistants or dental technicians. Arch. occup. environ. Health, 61(5), 329-333.

ETO, K., TOKUNAGA, H., ITAI, Y., TAKIZAWA, Y., & SUDA, H. (1988) [An autopsy of fetal Minamata disease which takes a long course.] Report presented at a Conference on the Comprehensive Study on Minamata Disease, 27 February, 1988, sponsored by the Environmental Agency, Japan (in Japanese).

EYBL, V., SYKORA, J., & MERTL, F. (1969) [Influence of sodium selenite, sodium tellurite and sodium sulphite on the retention and distribution of mercury in mice.] Arch. Toxikol., 25: 296-305 (in German with English summary).

FAN, P.L. (1987) Safety of amalgam. Cal. dent. Assoc. J., September: 34-36.

FARANT, J.P., BRISSETTE, D., MONCION, L., BIGRAS, L., & CHARTRAND, A. (1981) Improved cold-vapor atomic absorption technique for the microdetermination of total and inorganic mercury in biological samples. J. anal. Toxicol., 5: 47-51.

FAWER, R.F., DE RIBAUPIERRE, Y., GUILLEMIN, M.P., BERODE, M., & LOB, M. (1983) Measurement of hand tremor induced by industrial exposure to metallic mercury. Br. J. ind. Med., 40: 204-208.

FILLIASTRE, J.-P., DRUET, P., & MERY, J.-P. (1988) Proteinuric nephropathies associated with drugs and substances of abuse. In: Cameron, J.S. & Glassok, R.J. ed. The nephrotic syndrome, New York, Basel, Marcel Dekker Inc., pp. 697-742.

FINNE, K., GÖRANSSON, K., & WINCKLER, L. (1982) Oral lichen planus and contact allergy to mercury. Int. J. oral Surg., 11: 236-239.

FOA, V., CAIMI, L., AMANTE, L., ANTONINI, C., GATTINONI, A., TETTAMANTI, G., LOMBARDO, A., & GIULIANI, A. (1976) Patterns of some lysosomal enzymes in the plasma and of proteins in urine of workers exposed to inorganic mercury. Int. Arch. occup. environ. Health, 37: 115-124.

FOOTE, R.S. (1972) Mercury vapor concentrations inside buildings. Science, 177: 513-514.

FORZI, M., CASSITTO, M.G., BULGHERONI, C., & FOA, V. (1976) Psychological measures in workers occupationally exposed to mercury vapours. A validation study. In: Adverse effects of environmental chemicals and psychotoxic drugs, Amsterdam, Oxford, New York, Elsevier Science Publishers, Vol. 2, pp. 165-172.

FRIBERG, L. (1956) Studies on the accumulation, metabolism and excretion of inorganic mercury (Hg^{203}) after prolonged subcutaneous administration to rats. Acta pharmacol. toxicol., 12: 411-427.

FRIBERG, L. (1988) Quality assurance. In: Clarkson, T.W., Friberg, L., Nordberg, G.F., & Sager, P., ed. Biological monitoring of metals, New York, London, Plenum Press, pp. 103-126.

FRIBERG, L. & NYLANDER, M. (1987) [The release and uptake of metallic mercury vapour from amalgam.] In: Mercury/amalgam - health risks. Report by an expert group. Stockholm, National Board of Health and Welfare, Report series Socialstyrelsen Redovisar 1987, 10, pp. 65-79 (in Swedish with English summary).

FRIBERG, L. & VOSTAL, J. ed. (1972) [The release and uptake of metallic mercury vapour from amalgam.] In: [Mercury/amalgam - Health risks], Stockholm, National Board of Health and Welfare, pp. 65-79 (Report series Socialstyrelsen Redovisar 10) (in Swedish with English summary).

FRIBERG, L., SKOG, E., & WAHLBERG, J.E. (1961) Resorption of mercuric chloride and methyl mercury dicyandiamide in guinea-pigs through normal skin and through skin pre-treated with acetone, alkylarylsulphonate and soap. Acta dermatovenereol., **41**: 40-52.

FRIBERG, L., KULLMAN, L., LIND, B., & NYLANDER, M. (1986) [Mercury in the central nervous system in relation to amalgam fillings.] Laekartidningen, **83**: 519-522 (in Swedish).

FRYKHOLM, K.O. (1957) Mercury from dental amalgam. Its toxic and allergic effects and some comments on occupational hygiene. Acta odont. Scand., **22**: 1-108.

FUKATSU, A., BRENTJENS, J.R., KILLEN, P.D., KLEINMAN, H.K., MARTIN, G.R., & ANDRES, G.A. (1987) Studies on the formation of glomerular immune deposits in Brown Norway rats injected with mercuric chloride. Clin. Immunol. Immunopathol., **45**: 35-47.

FUKINO, H., HIRAI, M., MEI HSUEH, Y., MORIYASU, S., & YAMANE, Y. (1986) Mechanism of protection by zinc against mercuric chloride toxicity in rats: Effects of zinc and mercury on glutathionine metabolism. J. Toxicol. environ. Health, **19**: 75-89.

FUKUDA, K. (1971) Metallic mercury induced tremor in rabbits and mercury content of the central nervous system. Br. J. ind. Med., **28**: 308-311.

GALE, T.F. (1980) Cardiac and non-cardiac malformations produced by mercury in hamsters. Bull. environ. Contam. Toxicol., **25**: 726-732.

GALE, T.F. (1981) The embryotoxic response produced by inorganic mercury in different strains of hamsters. Environ. Res., **24**: 152-161.

GALE, T.F. (1984) The amelioration of mercury-induced embryotoxic effects by simultaneous treatment with zinc. Environ. Res., **35**: 405-411.

GALE, T.F. & FERM, V.H. (1971) Embryopathic effects of mercuric salts. Life Sci., **10**: 1341-1347.

GANSER, A.L. & KIRSCHNER, D.A. (1985) The interaction of mercurials with myelin: Comparison of *in vitro* and *in vivo* effects. Neurotoxicology, **6**(1): 63-78.

GAY, D.D., COX, R.D., & REINHARDT, J.W. (1979) Chewing releases mercury from fillings. Lancet, **8123**: 985-986.

GELLER, S.A. (1976) Subacute and chronic tissue reaction to metallic mercury: Two cases and a review of the literature. Mt Sinai J. Med., **43**: 534-541.

GLEICHMANN, E., PALS, S.T., ROLINK, A.G., RADASZKIEWICZ, T., & GLEICHMANN, H. (1984) Graft-versus-host reactions: clues to the etiopathology of a spectrum of immunological diseases. Immunol. Today, **5**(11): 324-332.

GONCHARUK, G.A. (1977) [Problems relating to occupational hygiene in women in production of mercury.] Gig. Tr. prof. Zabol., **5**: 17-20 (in Russian).

GORDON, H. (1981) Pregnancy in female dentists - a mercury hazard? In: Proceedings of the International Conference on Mercury Hazards in Dental Practice, Glasgow, 2-4 September, (Paper 31).

GOTELLI, C. (1989) Methylmercury in a gold mining region. Proc. Nat. Inst. Environm. Health Sci. (in print).

GOTELLI, C.A., ASTOLFI, E., COX, C., CERNICHIARI, E., & CLARKSON, T.W. (1985) Early biochemical effects of an organic mercury fungicide on infants: "dose makes the poison". Science, 227: 638-640.

GRITZKA, T.L. & TRUMP, B.F. (1968) Renal tubular lesions caused by mercuric chloride. Am. J. Pathol., 52(6): 1225-1277.

GRONKA, P.A., BOBKOSKIE, R.L., TOMCHICK, G.J., BACH, F., & RAKOW, A.B. (1970) Mercury vapor exposures in dental offices. J. Am. Dent. Assoc., 81: 923-925.

GRUENWEDEL, D.W. & DAVIDSON, N. (1966) Complexing and denaturation of DNA by methylmercuric hydroxide. J. mol. Biol., 21: 129-144.

HAHN, L.J., KLOIBER, R., VIMY, M.J., TAKAHASHI, Y., & LORSHEIDER, F.L. (1989) Dental "silver" tooth fillings: a source of mercury exposure revealed by whole-body image scan and tissue analysis. FASEB J., 3(14): 2641-2646.

HALBACH, S. & CLARKSON, T.W. (1978) Enzymatic oxidation of mercury vapors by erythrocytes. Biochem. Biophys. Acta, 523(2): 522-531.

HANDKE, J.L. & PRYOR, P. (1981) Health hazard evaluation report, Cincinnati, Ohio, National Institute for Occupational Safety and Health, 26 pp. (HHE 78-034-930).

HANSEN, J.C., KRISTENSEN, P., & AL-MASRI, S.N. (1981) Mercury/selenium interaction. A comparative study on pigs. Nord. vet. Med., 33: 57-64.

HANSEN, J.C., RESKE-NIELSEN, E., THORLACIUS-USSING, O., RUNGBY, J., & DANSHER, G. (1989) Distribution of dietary mercury in a dog. Quantitation and localization of total mercury in organs and central nervous system. Sci. tot. Environ., 78: 23-43.

HANSSON, M. (1986) [Changes in health after removal of toxic dental filling materials.] TF-BLADET, 1: 3-30 (in Swedish).

HARRIS, D., NICOLS, J.J., STARK, R., & HILL, K. (1978) The dental working environment and the risk of mercury exposure. J. Am. Dent. Assoc., 97: 811-815.

HATCH, W.R. & OTT, W.L. (1968) Determination of sub-microgram quantities of mercury by atomic absorption spectrophotometry. Anal. Chem., 40: 2085-2087.

HEIDAM, L.Z. (1984) Spontaneous abortions among dental assistants, factory workers, painters, and gardening workers: A follow up study. J. Epidemiol. community Health, 38: 149-155.

HEINTZE, U., EDWARDSSON, S., DERAND, T., & BIRKHED, D. (1983) Methylation of mercury from dental amalgam and mercuric chloride by oral streptococci in vitro. Scand. J. dent. Res., 91: 150-152.

HIRSCH, F., COUDERC, J., SAPIN, C., FOURNIE, G., & DRUET, P. (1982) Polyclonal effect of $HgCl_2$ in the rat, its possible role in an experimental autoimmune disease. Eur. J. Immunol., 12: 620-625.

HIRSHMAN, S.Z., FEINGOLD, M., & BOYLEN, G. (1963) Mercury in house paint as a cause of acrodynia: effect of therapy with N-acetyl-D,L-penicillamine. N. Engl. J. Med., 269: 889-893.

HOLT, D. & WEBB, M. (1986) The toxicity and teratogenicity of mercuric mercury in the pregnant rat. Arch. Toxicol., 58: 243-248.

HUBERLANT, J.M., ROELS, H., BUCHET, J.P., BERNARD, A., & LAUWERYS, R. (1983) Evaluation de l'exposition au mercure et de ses répercussions éventuelles sur la santé du personnel d'une trentaine de cabinets dentaires. Cah. Méd. Trav., 20(2): 109-127.

HUDSON, P.J., VOGT, R.L., BRONDUM, J., WITHERELL, L., MYERS, G., & PASCHAL, D.C. (1987) Elemental mercury exposure among children of thermometer plant workers. Pediatrics, 79(6): 935-938.

HULTMAN, P. & ENESTRÖM, S. (1987) The induction of immune complex deposits in mice by peroral and parenteral administration of mercuric chloride: Strain dependent susceptibility. Clin. exp. Immunol., 67: 283-292.

HULTMAN, P. & ENESTRÖM, S. (1988) Mercury induced antinuclear antibodies in mice: characterization and correlation with renal immune complex deposits. Clin. exp. Immunol., 71: 269-274.

HURSH, J.B. (1985) Particle coefficients of mercury (^{203}Hg) vapour between air and biological fluids. J. appl. Toxicol., 5: 327-332.

HURSH, J.B., CLARKSON, T.W., CHERIAN, M.G., VOSTAL, J.V., & MALLIE, R.V. (1976) Clearance of mercury (Hg-197, Hg-203) vapor inhaled by human subjects. Arch. environ. Health, 31: 302-309.

HURSH, J.B., GREENWOOD, M.R., CLARKSON, T.W., ALLEN, J., & DEMUTH, S. (1980) The effect of ethanol on the fate of mercury vapor inhaled by man. J. Pharmacol. exp. Ther., 214: 520-527.

HURSH, J.B., SICHAK, S.P., & CLARKSON, T.W. (1988) In vitro oxidation of mercury by the blood. Pharmacol. Toxicol., 63: 266-273.

HURSH, J.B., CLARKSON, T.W., MILES, E., & GOLDSMITH, L.A. (1989) Percutaneous absorption of mercury vapour by man. Arch. environ. Health, 44(2): 120-127.

IARC (1987) Overall evaluation of carcinogenicity: An updating of IARC Monographs Volumes 1 to 42, Lyon, International Agency for Research on Cancer, 440 pp. (IARC Monographs on the Evaluation of Carcinogenic Risk to Humans, Suppl. 7).

ICRP (1980) Metabolic data for mercury. Ann. int. Comm. rad. Prot., 30/Part 2, 4: 59-63.

IMURA, N. & NAGANUMA, A. (1978) Interaction of inorganic mercury and selenite in rabbit blood after intravenous administration. J. Pharm. Dyn., 1: 67-73.

INTERNATIONAL CLEARING-HOUSE FOR BIRTH DEFECTS MONITORING SYSTEM (1985) Annual report. Sidney, National Perinatal Statistics Unit, University of Sidney, 71 p. (ISSN 0743-5703).

ISHIHARA, N., URUSHIYAMA, K., & SUZUKI, T. (1977) Inorganic and organic mercury in blood, urine and hair in low level mercury vapour exposure. Int. Arch. occup. environ. Health, 40: 249-253.

JACOBS, M. & GOLDWATER, L.J. (1965) Absorption and excretion of mercury in man: VIII. Mercury exposure from house paint - a controlled study on humans. Arch. environ. Health, 11: 582-587.

JOHANSSON, E. & LINDH, U. (1987) Mercury in blood cells - altered elemental profiles. Toxic events in human exposure. Biol. Trace Elem. Res., 12: 309-321.

JOHNSON, S.L. & POND, W.G. (1974) Inorganic vs. organic Hg toxicity in growing rats: Protection by dietary Se but not Zn. Nutr. Rep. Int., 9(2): 135-147.

JOKSTAD, A. (1987) [Mercury exposure of dentists]. J. Norw. Dent. Assoc., 97: 498-507 (in Norwegian).

JOSELOW, M.M. & GOLDWATER, L.J. (1967) Absorption and excretion of mercury in man. XII. Relationship between urinary mercury and proteinuria. Arch. environ. Health, 15: 155.

JOSELOW, M.M., GOLDWATER, L.J., ALVAREZ, A., & HERNDON, J. (1968) Absorption and excretion of mercury in man. Arch. environ. Health, 17: 39-43.

JUANG, M.S. (1976) An electrophysiological study of the action of methylmercuric chloride and mercuric chloride on the sciatic nerve-sartorius muscle preparation of the frog. Toxicol. appl. Pharmacol., 37: 339-348.

JUGO, S. (1976) Retention and distribution of $^{203}HgCl_2$ in suckling and adult rats. Health Phys., 30: 240-241.

KANEMATSU, N., HARA, M., & KADA, T. (1980) Rec assay and mutagenicity studies on metal compounds. Mutat. Res., 77: 109-116.

KARK, P. (1979) Clinical and neurochemical aspects of inorganic mercury intoxication. In: Handbook of clinical neurology, Amsterdam, Oxford, New York, Elsevier Science Publishers, Vol. 36, pp. 147-197.

KAZANTZIS, G. (1978) The role of hypersensitivity and the immune response in influencing susceptibility to metal toxicity. Environ. Health Perspect., 25: 111-118.

KAZANTZIS, G. (1981) Role of cobalt, iron, lead, manganese, mercury, platinum, selenium, and titanium in carcinogenesis. Environ. Health Perspect., 40: 143-161.

KAZANTZIS, G. & LILLY, L.J. (1986) Mutagenic and carcinogenic effects of metals. In: Friberg, L., Nordberg, G.F., & Vouk, V., ed. Handbook on the toxicology of metals, Amsterdam, Oxford, New York, Elsevier Science Publishers, Vol. 1, pp. 319-390.

KAZANTZIS, G., SCHILLER, K.F.R., ASSCHER, A.W., & DREW, R.G. (1962) Albuminuria as the nephrotic syndrome following exposure to mercury and its compounds. Q. J. Med., 31(124): 403-418.

KELMAN, G.R. (1978) Notes and miscellanea: Urinary mercury excretion in dental personnel. Br. J. ind. Med., 35: 262-265.

KHAYAT, A. & DENCKER, L. (1982) Fetal uptake and distribution of metallic mercury vapor in the mouse: Influence of ethanol and aminotriazole. Biol. Res. Pregn., 3(1): 38-46.

KHAYAT, A. & DENCKER, L. (1983a) Whole body and liver distribution of inhaled mercury vapor in the mouse: Influence of ethanol and aminotriazole pretreatment. J. appl. Toxicol., 3: 66-74.

KHAYAT, A. & DENCKER, L. (1983b) Interactions between selenium and mercury in mice: Marked retention in the lung after inhalation of metallic mercury. Chem. biol. Interact., 46: 283-298.

KHAYAT, A. & DENCKER, L. (1984) Organ and cellular distribution of inhaled metallic mercury in the rat and marmoset monkey *(Callithrix jacchus):* Influence of ethyl alcohol pretreatment. Acta pharmacol. toxicol., 55: 145-152.

KIBUKAMUSOKE, J.W., DAVIES, D.R., & HUTT, M.S.R. (1974) Membranous nephropathy due to skin-lightening cream. Br. med. J., 2: 646-647.

KIMATA, H., SHINOMIYA, K., & MIKAWA, H. (1983) Selective enhancement of human IgE production in vitro by synergy of pokeweed mitogen and mercuric chloride. Clin. exp. Immunol., 53: 183-191.

KISHI, R., HASHIMOTO, K., SHIMIZU, S., & KOBAYASHI, M. (1978) Behavioral changes and mercury concentrations in tissues of rats exposed to mercury vapor. Toxicol. appl. Pharmacol., 46: 555-566.

KITAMURA, S., SUMINO, K., HAYAKAWA, K., & SHIBATA, T. (1976) Mercury content in human tissues from Japan. In: Nordberg, G.F., ed. Effects and dose-response relationships of toxic metals, Amsterdam, Oxford, New York, Elsevier Science Publishers, pp. 290-298.

KNEIP, T.J. & FRIBERG, L. (1986) Sampling and analytical methods. In: Friberg, L., Nordberg, G.F., & Vouk, V.B., ed. Handbook on the toxicology of metals, 2nd ed., Amsterdam, Oxford, New York, Elsevier Science Publishers, Vol. 1, pp. 36-67.

KNOFLACH, P., ALBINI, B., & WEISER, M.M. (1986) Autoimmune disease induced by oral administration of mercuric chloride in Brown-Norway rats. Toxicol. Pathol., 14(2): 188-193.

KOMSTA-SZUMSKA, E. & CHMIELNICKA, J. (1977) Binding of mercury and selenium in subcellular fractions of rat liver and kidneys following separate and joint administration. Arch. Toxicol., 38: 217-228.

KOSTA, L., BYRNE, A.R., & ZELENKO, V. (1975) Correlation between selenium and mercury in man following exposure to inorganic mercury. Nature, London, 254: 238-239.

KOSTIAL, K. & LANDEKA, M. (1975) The action of mercury ions on the release of acetylcholine from presynaptic nerve endings. Experientia, Basel, 31(7): 834-835.

KOSTIAL, K., KELLO, D., JUGO, S., RABAR, I., & MALJKOVIC, T. (1978) Influence of age on metal metabolism and toxicity. Environ. Health Perspect., 25: 81-86.

KOSTIAL, K., SIMONOVIC, I., RABAR, I., BLANUSA, M., & LANDEKA, M. (1983) Age and intestinal retention of mercury and cadmium in rats. Environ. Res., 31: 111-115.

KUSAKAWA, S. & HEINER, D.C. (1976) Elevated levels of immunoglobin E in the acute febrile mucocutaneous lymph node syndrome. Pediatr. Res., 10: 108-112.

LAMBETH, LONDON BOROUGH (1988) Mercury soaps and skin lightening cream. Directorate of environmental and consumer services, London.

LAMPERTI, A.A. & PRINTZ, R.H. (1973) Effects of mercuric chloride on the reproductive cycle of the female hamster. Biol. Reprod., 8: 378-387.

LAMPERTI, A.A. & PRINTZ, R.H. (1974) Localization, accumulation, and toxic effects of mercuric chloride on the reproductive axis of the female hamster. Biol. Reprod., 11: 180-186.

LAMPERTI, A. & NIEWENHUIS, R. (1976) The effects of mercury on the structure and function of the hypothalamo-pituitary axis in the hamster. Cell Tissue Res., 170: 315-324.

LANGAN, D.C., FAN, P.L., & HOOS, A.A. (1987) The use of mercury in dentistry: A critical review of the recent literature. J. Am. Dent. Assoc., 115: 867-880.

LANGOLF, G.D., CHAFFIN, D.B., HENDERSON, R., & WHITTLE, H.P. (1978)

Evaluation of workers exposed to elemental mercury using quantitative tests of tremor and neuromuscular functions. Am. Ind. Hyg. Assoc. J., **39**: 976-984.

LANGOLF, G.D., SMITH, P.J., HENDERSON, R., & WHITTLE, H.P. (1981) Measurements of neurological functions in the evaluations of exposure to neurotoxic agents. Ann. occup. Hyg., **24**(3): 293-296.

LANGWORTH, S. (1987) Renal function in workers exposed to inorganic mercury. In: Occupational health in the chemical industry: papers presented at the XXII ICOH congress, Sidney, Australia, 27 September-2 October 1987. Copenhagen, World Health Organization, p. 237.

LANGWORTH, S., ELINDER, C.-G., & ÅKESSON, A. (1988) Mercury exposure from dental fillings. I Mercury concentrations in blood and urine. Swed. dent. J., **12**: 69-70.

LAUWERYS, R., BERNARD, A., ROELS, H., BUCHET, J.P., GENNART, J.P., MAHIEU, P., & FOIDART, J.M. (1983) Anti-laminin antibodies in workers exposed to mercury vapour. Toxicol. Lett., **17**: 113-116.

LAUWERYS, R., ROELS, H., GENET, P., TOUSSAINT, G., BOUCKAERT, A., & DE COOMAN, S. (1985) Fertility of male workers exposed to mercury vapor or to manganese dust: A questionnaire study. Am. J. ind. Med., **7**: 171-176.

LAUWERYS, R., BONNIER, C., EVRARD, P., GENNART, J., & BERNARD, A. (1987) Prenatal and early postnatal intoxication by inorganic mercury resulting from the maternal use of mercury-containing soap. Hum. Toxicol., **6**: 253-256.

LAVSTEDT, S. & SUNDBERG, H. (1989) [Medical diagnosis and disease symptoms related to amalgam fillings.] Tandläkartidningen, **3**: 81-88 (in Swedish).

LEE, I.P. & DIXON, R.L. (1975) Effects of mercury on spermatogenesis studied by velocity sedimentation cell separation and serial mating. J. Pharmacol. exp. Ther., **194**(1): 171-181.

LEE, S.A. (1984) Health hazard evaluation report, Cincinnati, Ohio, National Institute for Occupational Safety and Health, 10 pp. (HETA 83-338-1399).

LEONARD, A., JACQUET, P., & LAUWERYS, R.R. (1983) Mutagenicity and teratogenicity of mercury compounds. Mutat. Res., **114**: 1-18.

LEVIN, M., JACOBS, J., & POLOS, P.G. (1988) Acute mercury poisoning and mercurial pneumonitis from gold ore purification. Chest, **94**: 554-556.

LEVINE, S.P., CAVENDER, G.D., LANGOLF, G.D., & ALBERS, J.W. (1982) Elemental mercury exposure: peripheral neurotoxicity. Br. J. ind. Med., **39**: 136-139.

LIND, B,. FRIBERG, L., & NYLANDER, M. (1988) Preliminary studies on methylmercury biotransformation and clearance in the brain of primates: II. Demethylation of mercury in brain. J. Trace Elem. exp. Med., **1**: 49-56.

LINDBERG, S., STOKES, P., GOLDBERG, E., & WREN, C. (1987) Group Report: Mercury. In: Hutchinson, T.W. & Meemz, K.M. ed. Lead, mercury, cadmium and arsenic in the environment, New York, Chichester, Brisbane, Toronto, John Wiley & Sons, pp. 17-34 (Scope 31).

LINDQVIST, K.J., MAKENE, W.J., SHABA, J.K., & NANTULYA, V. (1974) Immunofluorescence and electron microscopic studies of kidney biopsies from patients with nephrotic syndrome, possibly induced by skin lightening creams containing mercury. East Afr. med. J., **51**: 168-169.

LINDQVIST, O, JERNELOV, A., JOHANNSON, K., & RODHE, R. (1984) Mercury in the swedish environment: global and local sources. Solna, National Environmental Protection Board, 105 pp. (Report No. 1816).

LINDSTEDT, G., GOTTBERG, I., HOLMGREN, B., JONSSON, T., & KARLSSON, G. (1979) Individual mercury exposure of chloralkali workers and its relation to blood and urinary mercury levels. Scand. J. Work Environ. Health, **5**: 59-69.

LINKE, W.F. (1958) Inorganic and metal-organic compounds, New York, Van Nostrand Reinhold Company Inc.

LUNDBORG, M., LIND, B., & CAMNER, P. (1984) Ability of rabbit alveolar macrophages to dissolve metals. Exp. Lung Res., **7**: 11-22.

MABILLE, V., ROELS, H., JACQUET, P., LEONARD, A., & LAUWERYS, R. (1984) Cytogenetic examination of leucocytes of workers exposed to mercury vapour. Int. Arch. occup. environ. Health, **53**: 257-260.

MCCAMMON, C.S., Jr, EDWARDS, S.L., DELON HULL, R., & WOODFIN, W.J. (1980) A comparison of four personal sampling methods for the determination of mercury vapor. Am. Ind. hyg. Assoc. J., **41**: 528-531.

MCFARLAND, R.B. & REIGEL, H. (1978) Chronic mercury poisoning from a single brief exposure. J. occup. Med., **20**(8): 532-534.

MACKERT, J.R., Jr, (1987) Factors affecting estimation of dental amalgam mercury exposure from measurements of mercury vapor levels in intra-oral and expired air. J. dent. Res., **66**(12): 1775-1780.

MCNERNEY, J.J, BUSECK, P.R., & HANSON, R.C. (1972) Mercury detection by means of thin gold films. Science, **178**: 611-612.

MAGNUSSON, J. & RAMEL, C. (1986) Genetic variation in the susceptibility to mercury and other metal compounds in *Drosophila melanogaster*. Teratog. Carcinog. Mutagen., **6**: 289-192.

MAGOS, L. (1971) Selective atomic-absorption determination of inorganic mercury and methylmercury in undigested biological samples. Analyst, **96**: 847-853.

MAGOS, L. & CLARKSON, T.W. (1972) Atomic absorption determination of total, inorganic and organic mercury in blood. J. Assoc. Off. Anal. Chem., 5(5): 966-971.

MAGOS, L., WEBB, M., & BUTLER, W.H. (1974) The effect of cadmium pretreatment on the nephrotoxic action and kidney uptake of mercury in male and female rats. Br. J. exp. Pathol., 55: 589-594.

MAGOS, L., HALBACH, S., & CLARKSON, T.W. (1978) Role of catalase in the oxidation of mercury vapor. Biochem. Pharmacol., 27: 1373-1377.

MAGOS, L., SPARROW, S., & SNOWDEN, R. (1982) The comparative renotoxicology of phenylmercury and mercuric chloride. Arch. Toxicol., 50: 133-139.

MAGOS, L., CLARKSON, T.W., & HUDSON, A.R. (1984) Differences in the effects of selenite and biological selenium on the chemical form and distribution of mercury after the simultaneous administration of $HgCl_2$ and selenium to rats. J. Pharmacol. exp. Ther., 228(2): 478-483.

MAGOS, L., BROWN, A.W., SPARROW, S., BAILEY, E., SNOWDEN, R.T., & SKIPP, W.R. (1985) The comparative toxicology of ethyl- and methyl-mercury. Arch. Toxicol., 57: 260-267.

MAGOS, L., CLARKSON, T.W., SPARROW, S., & HUDSON, A.R. (1987) Comparison of the protection given by selenite, selenomethionine and biological selenium against the renotoxicity of mercury. Arch. Toxicol., 60: 422-426.

MANALIS, R.S. & COOPER, G.P. (1975) Evoked transmitter release increased by inorganic mercury at frog neuromuscular junction. Nature, London, 257: 690-691.

MARAFANTE, E., LUNDBORG, M., VAHTER, M., & CAMNER, P. (1987) Dissolution of two arsenic compounds by rabbit alveolar macrophages in vitro. Fundam. appl. Toxicol., 8: 382-388.

MARZULLI, F.N. & BROWN, D.W.C. (1972) Potential systemic hazards of topically applied mercurials. J. Soc. cosmet. Chem., 23: 875-886.

MATHESON, D.S., CLARKSON, T.W., & GELFAND, E.W. (1980) Mercury toxicity (acrodynia) induced by long-term injection of gammaglobulin. J. Pediatr., 97(1): 153-155.

MATTIUSSI, R., ARMELI, G., & BAREGGI, V. (1982) Statistical study of the correlation between mercury exposure (TWA) and urinary mercury concentrations in chloralkali workers. Am. J. ind. Med., 3: 335-339.

MENGEL, H. & KARLOG, O. (1980) Studies on the interaction and distribution of selenite, mercuric, methoxyethyl mercuric and methyl mercuric chloride in rats. II. Analysis of the soluble proteins and the precipitates of liver and kidney homogenates. Acta pharmacol. toxicol., 46: 25-31.

MILLER, E.G., PERRY, W.L., & WAGNER, M.J. (1987) Prevalence of mercury hypersensitivity in dental students. J. prosthet. Dent., 58: 235-237.

MILLER, J.M., CHAFFIN, D.B., & SMITH, R.G. (1975) Subclinical psychomotor and neuromuscular changes in workers exposed to inorganic mercury. Am. Ind. Hyg. Assoc. J., 36: 725-733.

MINAGAWA, K., HIRASAWA, F., HOZUMI, S., CHUANG, K., & TAKIZAWA, Y. (1979) [Rapid determinations of total mercury and methylmercury in biological samples.] Akita J. Med., 5: 263-271 (in Japanese with English summary).

MIRTSCHEWA, J., NÜRNBERGER, W., HALLMANN, B., STILLER-WINKLER, R., & GLEICHMANN, E. (1987) Genetically determined susceptibility of mice to $HgCl_2$-induced antinuclear antibodies (ANA) and glomerulo-nephritis. Immunobiology, 175: 323-324.

MIYAMA, T. & SUZUKI, T. (1971) Release of mercury from organs and breakage of carbon-mercury bond in tissues due to formalin fixation. Jpn. J. ind. Health, 13(6): 56-57.

MIYAMOTO, M.D. (1983) Hg^{2+} causes neurotoxicity at an intracellular site following entry through Na and Ca channels. Brain Res., 267: 375-379.

MOLIN, M., BERGMAN, B., MARKLUND, S.L., SCHÜTZ, A., & SKERFVING, S. (1990) Mercury, selenium and glutathione peroxidase before and after amalgam removal in man. Acta Odontol. Scand., 48(3): 189-202.

MOLLER-MADSEN, B. & DANSCHER, G. (1986) Localization of mercury in CNS of the rat. Environ. Res., 41: 29-43.

MORIMOTO, K., IIJIMA, S., & KOIZUMI, A. (1982) Selenite prevents the induction of sister-chromatid exchanges by methylmercury and mercuric chloride in human whole-blood cultures. Mutat. Res., 102: 183-192.

MÖRNER, S. & NILSSON, T. (1986) [Mercury discharge from crematories in Gothenburg], City of Gothenburg, Environmental and Health Protection Agency (Report 1986.1) (in Swedish).

MORROW, P.E., GIBB, F.R., & JOHNSON, L. (1964) Clearance of insoluble dust from the lower respiratory tract. Health Phys., 10: 543-555.

MOTTET, K. & BURBACHER, T. M. (1988) Preliminary studies on methylmercury biotransformation and clearance in the brain of primates: I. Experimental design and general observations J. Trace Elem. exp. Med., 1: 41-47.

MüLLER, H.,VON, SCHUBERT, H., & VERBEEK, W. (1980) [Report on the relationship between Hg concentration in urine and blood and Hg concentration in workroom air.] Arbeitsmed. Sozialmed. Präventivmed., 15: 64-67 (in German with English summary).

MURAMATSU, Y. & PARR, R.M. (1985) Survey of currently available reference materials for use in connection with the determination of trace elements in biological and environmental materials. Vienna, International Atomic Energy Agency (Report No. IAEA/RL/128).

MUTTI, A., LUCERTINI, S., FORNARI, M., FRANCHINI, I., BERNARD, A., ROELS, H., & LAUWERYS, R. (1985) Urinary excretion of a brush border antigen revealed by monoclonal antibodies in subjects occupationally exposed to heavy metals. In: Proceedings of the International Conference on Heavy Metals in the Environment, Luxembourg, Commission of the European Communities, Vol. 1, pp. 565-567.

NAGANUMA, A. & IMURA, N. (1980) Bis(methylmercuric) selenide as a reaction product from methylmercury and selenite in rabbit blood. Res. Commun. chem. Pathol. Pharmacol., 27(1): 163-173.

NAKAAKI, K., FUKABORI, S., & TADA, O. (1975) [An experimental study on inorganic mercury vapour exposure.] J. Sci. Labour, 51(12): 705-716 (in Japanese with English summary).

NAKAAKI, K., FUKABORI, S., & TADA, O. (1978) On the evaluation of mercury exposure. J. sci. Labour, 54: 1-8.

NAKADA, S., NOMOTO, A., & IMURA, N. (1980) Effect of methylmercury and inorganic mercury on protein synthesis in mammalian cells. Ecotoxicol. environ. Saf., 4: 184-190.

NAKAYAMA, H., NIKI, F., SHONO, M., & HADA, S. (1983) Mercury exanthem. Contact dermatitis, 9: 411-417.

NALEWAY, C., SAKAGUCHI, R., MITCHELL, E., MULLER, T., AYER, W.A., & HEFFERREN, J.J. (1985) Urinary mercury levels in US dentists, 1975-1983: Review of Health Assessment Program. J. Am. Dent. Assoc., 111: 37-42.

NATIONAL ACADEMY OF SCIENCES (1978) An assessment of mercury in the environment, Washington, DC, National Academy of Sciences, National Research Council.

NEWTON, D. & FRY, F.A. (1978) The retention and distribution of radioactive mercuric oxide following accidental inhalation. Ann. occup. Hyg., 21: 21-32.

NILSEN, A., NYBERG, K., & CAMNER, P. (1988) Intraphagosomal pH in alveolar macrophages after phagocytosis *in vivo* and *in vitro* of fluorescein-labeled yeast particles. Exp. Lung Res., 13: 197-207.

NILSSON, B. & NILSSON, B. (1986a) Mercury in dental practice. I. The working environment of dental personnel and their exposure to mercury vapor. Swed. dent. J., 10: 1-14.

NILSSON, B. & NILSSON, B. (1986b) Mercury in dental practice. II. Urinary mercury excretion in dental personnel. Swed. dent. J., 10: 221-232.

NISHIYAMA, S., TAGUCHI, T., & ONOSAKA, S. (1987) Induction of zinc-thionein by estradiol and protective effects on inorganic mercury-induced renal toxicity. Biochem. Pharmacol., 36(20): 3387-3391.

NIXON, G.S., WHITTLE, C.A., & WOODFIN, A. (1981) Mercury levels in dental surgeries and dental personnel. Br. dent. J., **151**: 149-154.

NORDLIND, K. (1985) Binding and uptake of mercuric chloride in human lymphoid cells. Int. Arch. Allergy appl. Immunol., **77**: 405-408.

NORDLIND, K. & HENZE, A. (1984) Stimulating effect of mercuric chloride and nickel sulfate on DNA synthesis of thymocytes and peripheral blood lymphocytes in children. Int. Arch. Allergy appl. Immunol., **73**: 162-165.

NORTH AMERICAN CONTACT DERMATITIS GROUP (1973) Epidemiology of contact dermatitis in North America, 1972. Arch. Dermatol., **108**: 537-540.

NRIAGU, J.O. (1979) The biogeochemistry of mercury in the environment, Amsterdam, Oxford, New York, Elsevier Science Publishers.

NYGAARD, S.F. & HANSEN, J.C. (1978) Mercury-selenium interaction at concentrations of selenium and of mercury vapours as prevalent in nature. Bull. environ. Contam. Toxicol., **20**: 20-23.

NYLANDER, M., FRIBERG, L., & LIND, B. (1987) Mercury concentrations in the human brain and kidneys in relation to exposure from dental amalgam fillings. Swed. dent. J., **11**: 179-187.

NYLANDER, M., FRIBERG, L., LIND, B., & AAKERBERG, S. (1988) Effects of breathing patterns on mercury release. In: Clarkson, T.W., Friberg, L., Nordberg, G.F., & Sager, P.R., ed. Biological monitoring of toxic metals, New York, London, Plenum Press, pp. 263-264.

NYLANDER, M., FRIBERG, L., EGGLESTON, D., & BJÖRKMAN, L. (1989) Mercury accumulation in tissues from dental staff and controls in relation to exposure. Swed. dent. J., **13**: 235-243.

OBERLY, T.J., PIPER, C.E., & MCDONALD, D.S. (1982) Mutagenicity of metals in the L5178Y mouse lymphoma assay. J. Toxicol. environ. Health, **9**: 367-376.

OGATA, M. & MEGURO, T. (1986) Foetal distribution of inhaled mercury vapor in normal and acatalasaemic mice. Physiol. Chem. Phys. med. NMR, **18**: 165-170.

OGATA, M., KENMOTSU, K., HIROTA, N., MEGURO, T., & AIKOH, H. (1987) Reduction of mercuric ion and exhalation of mercury in acatalasemic and normal mice. Arch. environ. Health, **42**(1): 26-30.

OKAMOTO, K., (1988) Biological reference materials from the National Institute for Environmental Studies (Japan). Fresenius Z. anal. Chem., **332**: 524-527.

OLSSON, B. & BERGMAN, M. (1987) Letter to the Editor. J. dent. Res., **66**(7): 1288-1291.

OLSTAD, M.L., HOLLAND, R.I., WANDEL, N., & HENSTEN PETTERSEN, A. (1987) Correlation between amalgam restorations and mercury concentrations in urine. J. dent. Res., **66**(6): 1179-1182.

ORLOWSKI, J.P. & MERCER, R.D. (1980) Urine mercury levels in Kawasaki disease. Pediatrics, 66(4): 633-636.

OTT, K.H.R., LOH, F., KRÖNCKE, A., SCHALLER, K.-H., VALENTIN, H., & WELTLE, D. (1984) [Mercury burden due to amalgam fillings.] Dtsch. Zahnärztl. Z., 39: 199-205 (in German with English summary).

PACYNA, J.M. (1987) Atmospheric emissions of arsenic, cadmium, lead and mercury from high temperature processes in power generation and industry. In: Hutchinson, T.C. & Meema, K.M. ed. Lead, mercury, cadmium and arsenic in the environment, New York, Chichester, Brisbane, Toronto, John Wiley & Sons, pp. 69-88 (Scope 31).

PAN, S.K., IMURA, N., YAMAMURA, Y., YOSHIDA, M., & SUZUKI, T. (1980) Urinary methylmercury excretion in persons exposed to elemental mercury vapor. Tohoku J. exp. Med., 130: 91-95.

PARIZEK, J. & OSTADALOVA, I. (1967) The protective effect of small amounts of selenite in sublimate intoxication. Experientia, Basel, 23(2): 142-143.

PARIZEK, J., OSTADALOVA, I., KALOUSKOVA, J., BABICKY, A., PAVLIK, L., & BIBR, B. (1971) Effect of mercuric compounds on the maternal transmission of selenium in the pregnant and lactating rat. J. Reprod. Fertil., 25: 157-170.

PARR, R.M., MURAMATSU, Y., & CLEMENTS, S.A. (1987) Survey and evaluation of available biological reference materials for trace element analysis. Fresenius Z. anal. Chem., 326: 601-608.

PARR, R.M., SCHELENZ, R., & BALLESTRA, S. (1988) IAEA biological reference materials. Fresenius Z. anal. Chem., 332: 518-523.

PATON, G.R. & ALLISON, A.C. (1972) Chromosome damage in human cell cultures induced by metal salts. Mutat. Res., 16: 332-336.

PATTERSON, J.E., WEISSBERG, B.G., & DENNISON, P.J. (1985) Mercury in human breath from dental amalgams. Bull. environ. Contam. Toxicol., 34: 459-468.

PELLETIER, L., PASQUIER, R., HIRSH, F., SAPIN, C., & DRUET, P. (1986) Autoreactive T cells in mercury-induced autoimmune disease: in vitro demonstration. J. Immunol., 137(8): 2548-2554.

PELLETIER, L., PASQUIER, R., VIAL, M.C., MANDET, C., MOUTIER, R., SALOMON, J.C., & DRUET, P. (1987a) Mercury-induced autoimmune glomerulonephritis: Requirement for T-cells. Nephrol. Dial. Transplant., 1: 211-218.

PELLETIER, L., GALCERAN, M., PASQUIER, R., RONCO, P., VERROUST, P., BARIETY, J., & DRUET, P. (1987b) Down modulation of Heymann's nephritis by mercuric chloride. Kidney Int., 32: 227-232.

PELLETIER, L., PASQUIER, R., ROSSERT, J., & DRUET, P. (1987c) $HgCl_2$ induces nonspecific immunosuppression in Lewis rats. Eur. J. Immunol., 17: 49-54.

PELLETIER, L., PASQUIER, R., GUETTIER, C., VIAL, M.C., MANDET, C., NOCHY, D., & DRUET, P. (1988a) $HgCl_2$ induces T and B cells to proliferate and differentiate in BN rats. Clin. exp. Immunol., 71: 336-342.

PELLETIER, L., PASQUIER, R., ROSSERT, J., VIAL, M.C., MANDET, C., & DRUET, P. (1988b) Autoreactive T-cells in mercury-induced autoimmunity. Ability to induce the autoimmune disease. J. Immunol., 140(3): 750-754.

PELLETIER, L., ROSSERT, J., PASQUIER, R., VILLARROYA, H., BELAIR, M.F., VIAL, M.C., ORIOL, R., & DRUET, P. (1988c) Effect of $HgCl_2$ on experimental allergic encephalomyelitis in Lewis rats. $HgCl_2$ induces down modulation of the disease. Eur. J. Immunol., 18: 243-247.

PENZER, V. (1986) Amalgam toxicity: grand deception. Int. J. Orthod., 24: 21-24.

PETER, F. & STRUNC, G. (1984) Semiautomated analysis for mercury in whole blood, urine and hair by on-stream generation of cold vapor. Clin. Chem., 30(6): 893-895.

PEZEROVIC, Dz., NARANCSIK, P., & GAMULIN, S. (1981) Effects of mercury bichloride on mouse kidney polyribosome structure and function. Arch. Toxicol., 48: 167-172.

PIIKIVI, L. & HANNINEN, H. (1989) Subjective symptoms and psychological performance of chlorin-alkali workers. Scand. J. Work. Environ. Health, 15: 69-74.

PIIKIVI, L. & TOLONEN, U. (1989) EEG findings in chlor-alkali workers subjected to low long term exposure to mercury vapour. Brit. J. ind. Med., 46: 370-375.

PIIKIVI, L., HANNINEN, H., MARTELIN, T., & MANTERE, P. (1984) Psychological performance and long-term exposure to mercury vapors. Scand. J. Work environ. Health, 10: 35-41.

PIOTROWSKI, J.K., TROJANOWSKA, B., & MOGILNICKA, E.M. (1975) Excretion kinetics and variability in urinary mercury in workers exposed to mercury vapor. Internat. Arch. occup. environ. Health, 35: 245-256.

POLAK, L., BARNES, J.M., & TURK, J.L. (1968) The genetic control of contact sensitization to inorganic metal compounds in guinea-pigs. Immunology, 14: 707-711.

POPESCU, H.I., NEGRU, L., & LANCRANJAN, I. (1979) Chromosome aberrations induced by occupational exposure to mercury. Arch. environ. Health., 34(6): 461-463.

PRICE, J.H. & WISSEMAN, C.L. (1977) Hazard evaluation and technical assistance report, Cincinnati, Ohio, National Institute for Occupational Safety and Health, 17 pp. (TA 77-52).

PRITCHARD, J.G., McMULLIN, J.F., & SIKONDARI, A.H. (1982) The prevalence of high levels of mercury in dentists' hair. Br. dent. J., **153**: 333-336.

PROUVOST-DANON, A., ABADIE, A., SAPIN, C., BAZIN, H., & DRUET, P. (1981) Induction of IgE synthesis and potentiation of anti-ovalbumin IgE antibody response by $HgCl_2$ in the rat. J. Immunol., 126(2): 699-702.

RAHOLA, T., HATTULA, T., KOROLAINEN, A., & MIETTINEN, J.K. (1973) Elimination of free and protein-bound ionic mercury ($^{203}Hg^{2+}$) in man. Ann. clin. Res., **5**: 214-219.

RAMEL, C. (1972) Genetic effects. In: Friberg, L. & Vostal, J., ed. Mercury in the environment, Cleveland, Ohio, CRC Press, Chapter 9, pp. 169-181.

RASBERRY, S.D. (1987) Biological reference materials from the US National Bureau of Standards - an update. Fresenius Z. anal. Chem., **326**: 609-612.

REINHARDT, J.W., KAI, CHIU CHAN, & SCHULEIN, T.M. (1983) Mercury vaporization during amalgam removal. J. prosthet. Dent., **50**(1): 62-64.

REUTER, R., TRESSARS, G., VOHR, H.-W., GLEICHMANN, E., & LÜHRMANN, R. (1989) Mercuric chloride induces autoantibodies to small nuclear ribonucleoprotein in susceptible mice. Proc. Natl Acad. Sci. (USA), **86**: 237-241.

RICE, D.C. (1989) Brain and tissue levels of mercury after chronic methylmercury exposure in the monkey. J. Toxicol. environ. Health, **27**: 189-190.

RICHARDS, J.M. & WARREN, P.J. (1985) Mercury vapour released during the removal of old amalgam restorations. Br. dent. J., **159**: 231-232.

RIZZO, A.M. & FURST, A. (1972) Mercury teratogenesis in the rat. Proc. West. Pharmacol. Soc., **15**: 52-54.

ROBINSON, G.C.J., BALAZS, T., & EGOROV, I.K. (1986) Mercuric chloride-, gold sodium thiomalate-, and D-penicillamine-induced antinuclear antibodies in mice. Toxicol. appl. Pharmacol., **86**: 159-169.

ROBISON, S.H., CANTONI, O., & COSTA, M. (1984) Analysis of metal-induced DNA lesions and DNA-repair replication in mammalian cells. Mutat. Res., **131**: 173-181.

ROELS, H., LAUWERYS, R., BUCHET, J.P., BERNARD, A., BARTHELS, A., OVERSTEYNS, M., & GAUSSIN, J. (1982) Comparison of renal function and psychomotor performance in workers exposed to elemental mercury. Int. Arch. occup. environ. Health, **50**: 77-93.

ROELS, H., GENNART, J.-P., LAUWERYS, R., BUCHET, J.-P., MALCHAIRE, J., & BERNARD, A. (1985) Surveillance of workers exposed to mercury vapour: Validation of a previously proposed biological threshold limit value for mercury concentration in urine. Am. J. ind. Med., **7**: 45-71.

ROELS, H., ABDELADIM, S., CEULEMANS, E., & LAUWERYS, R. (1987) Relationships between the concentrations of mercury in air and in blood or urine in workers exposed to mercury vapour. Ann. occup. Hyg., 31(2): 135-145.

ROMAN-FRANCO, A.A., TURIELLO, M., ALBINI, B., OSSI, E., MILGROM, F., & ANDRES, G.A. (1978) Anti-basement membrane antibodies and antigen-antibody complexes in rabbits injected with mercuric chloride. Clin. Immunol. Immunopathol., 9: 464-481.

ROSENMAN, K.D., VALCIUKAS, J.A., GLICKMAN, L., MEYERS, B.R., CINOTTI, A. (1986) Sensitive indicators of inorganic mercury toxicity. Arch. environ. Health, 41(4): 208-215.

ROSSI, L.C., CLEMENTE, G.F., & SANTARONI, G. (1976) Mercury and selenium distribution in a defined area and in its population. Arch. environ. Health, 160-165.

ROWLAND, I.R., GRASSO, P., & DAVIES, M.J. (1975) The methylation of mercuric chloride by human intestinal bacteria. Experentia, Basel, 31(9): 1064-1065.

ROZALSKI, M. & WIERZBICKI, R. (1983) Effect of mercuric chloride on cultured rat fibroblasts: Survival, protein biosynthesis and binding of mercury to chromatin. Biochem. Pharmacol., 32(13): 2124-2126.

RUDZKI, E. (1979) Occupational dermatitis among health service workers. Derm. Beruf Umwelt, 27(4): 112.

SAPIN, C., DRUET, E., & DRUET, P. (1977) Induction of anti-glomerular basement membrane antibodies in the Brown-Norway rat by mercuric chloride. Clin. exp. Immunol., 28: 173-179.

SAPIN, C., HIRSH, F., DELAPORTE, J.P., BAZIN, H., & DRUET, P. (1984) Polyclonal IgE increase after $HgCl_2$ injections in BN and LEW rats: a genetic analysis. Immunogenetics, 20: 227-236.

SAPOTA, A., PIOTROWSKI, J., & BARANSKI, B. (1974) Levels of metallothionein in the fetuses and tissues of pregnant rats exposed to mercury vapors. Med. Pr., 25: 129-136 (in Polish) (The original is not available. Quoted from US Public Health Service, Agency for Toxic Substances and Disease Registry, 1989).

SCHIELE, R. (1988) [Statement on uptake of mercury from amalgam]. In: Institut der Deutschen Zahnärzte (IDZ), ed. [Amalgam - for and against], Köln, Deutscher Arzte-Verlag, pp. 123-133 (in German).

SCHIELE, R., SCHALLER, K.-H., & GROBE, T. (1979) [Studies of persons occupationally exposed to mercury.] Arbeitsmed. Sozialmed. Präventivmed., 10: 226-229 (in German).

SCHNEIDER, M. (1974) An environmental study of mercury contamination in dental offices. J. Am. Dent. Assoc., 89: 1092-1098.

SCHROEDER, H. & MITCHENER, M. (1975) Life-term effects of mercury, methylmercury, and nine other trace metals on mice. J. Nutr., 105: 452-458.

SCHUCKMANN, F. (1979) Study of preclinical changes in workers exposed to inorganic mercury in chloralkali plants. Int. Arch. occup. environ. Health, 44: 193-200.

SCHÖPF, E., SCHULZ, K.H., & ISENSEE, I. (1969) [Investigations on lymphocyte transformation in mercury sensitivity. Nonspecific transformation due to mercury compounds.] Arch. klin. exp. Dermatol., 234: 420-433 (in German with English summary).

SECO, J.M. (1987) Big mercury deposit found in Spain. Financ. Times, Oct. 30.

SHAPIRO, I.M., CORNBLATH, D.R., SUMNER, A.J., UZZELL, B., SPITZ, L.K., SHIP, I.I., & BLOCH, P. (1982) Neurophysiological and neuropsychological function in mercury-exposed dentists. Lancet, I: 1147-1150.

SIBBET, D.J., MOYER, R., & MILLY, G. (1972) Emission of mercury from latex paint. Proceedings of the Division of Water, Air, and Waste Chemistry, Boston, American Chemical Society, pp. 20-26.

SIBLERUD, R.L. (1988) The relationship between dental amalgam and health. Dissertation, Colorado State University (partial fulfillment of a Ph.D. degree requirement in physiology).

SIKORSKI, R., JUSZKIEWICZ, T., PASZKOWSKI, T., & SZPRENGIER-JUSZKIEWICZ, T. (1987) Women in dental surgeries: Reproductive hazards in occupational exposure to metallic mercury. Int. Arch. occup. environ. Health, 59: 551-557.

SINCLAIR, P.M., TURNER, P.R.C., & JOHNS, R.B. (1980) Mercury levels in dental students and faculty measured by neutron activation analysis. J. prosthet. Dent., 43: 581-585.

SINGER, R., VALCIUKAS, J.A., & ROSENMAN, K.D. (1987) Peripheral neurotoxicity in workers exposed to inorganic mercury compounds. Arch. environ. Health, 42: 181-184.

SKARE, I. (1972) Microdetermination of mercury in biological samples. Part III. Automated determination of mercury in urine, fish and blood samples. Analyst, 97: 148-155.

SKARE, I. & ENGQVIST, A. (1986) [Mercury in air. Part I. Evaluation of solid adsorbents for exposure monitoring of mercury vapour], Solna, National Institute of Occupational Health, 47 pp. (Arbete och Hälsa 1986:38) (in Swedish with English summary).

SKERFVING, S. (1988) Mercury in women exposed to methylmercury through fish consumption, and in their newborn babies and breast milk. Bull. environ. Contam. Toxicol., 41: 475-482.

SKERFVING, S. & BERLIN, M. (1985) [Nordic expert group for limit value documentation 59. Inorganic mercury], Solna, National Institute of Occupational Health, 80 pp. (Arbete och Hälsa) (in Swedish with English summary).

SKERFVING, S. & VOSTAL, J. (1972) Symptoms and signs of intoxication. In: Friberg, L. & Vostal, J., ed. Mercury in the environment, Cleveland, Ohio, CRC Press, pp. 93-107.

SKOG, E. & WAHLBERG, J.E. (1964) A comparative investigation of the percutaneous absorption of metal compounds in the guinea-pig by means of the radioactive isotopes: ^{31}Cr, ^{36}Co, ^{63}Zn, ^{110m}Cd, ^{203}Hg. J. invest. Dermatol., 43: 187-192.

SKUBA, A.R.N. (1984) Survey for mercury vapour in Manitoba dental offices (Summer 1983). Can. Dent. Assoc. J., (7): 517-522.

SLEMR, F., HEINZ, G.H., CAMARDESE, M.B., HILL, E.F., MOORE, J.F., & MURRAY, H.C. (1981) Latitudinal distribution of mercury over the Atlantic Ocean. J. geophys. Res., 86: 1159-1166.

SMITH, P.J., LANGOLF, G.D., & GOLDBERG, J. (1983) Effects of occupational exposure to elemental mercury on short term memory. Br. J. ind. Med., 40: 413-419.

SMITH, R.G., VORWALD, A.J., PATIL, L.S., & MOONEY, T.F., Jr, (1970) Effects of exposure to mercury in the manufacture of chlorine. Am. Ind. Hyg. Assoc. J., 31: 687-700.

SNAPP, K.R., BOYER, D.B., PETERSON, L.C., & SVARE, C.W. (1989) The contribution of dental amalgam to mercury in blood. J. dent. Res., 68: 780-785.

SOS (1987) [Mercury/amalgam - Health risks.] Stockholm, National Board of Health and Welfare (Report by the LEK-Committee) (in Swedish with English summary).

STEFFEK, A.J., CLAYTON, R., SIEW, C., & VERRUSIO, A.C. (1987) Effects of elemental mercury vapor exposure on pregnant Sprague-Dawley rats. J. dent. Res., 66: 239.

STENMAN, E. & BERGMAN, M. (1989) Hypersensitivity reactions to dental materials in a referred group of patients. Scand. J. dent. Res., 97: 76-83.

STEWART, W.K., GUIRGIS, H.A., SANDERSON, J., & TAYLOR, W. (1977) Urinary mercury excretion and proteinuria in pathology laboratory staff. Br. J. ind. Med., 34: 26-31.

STOCK, A. (1939) [Chronic mercury and amalgam intoxication.] Zahnärztl. Rundsch., 10: 371-377, 403-700 (in German).

STONARD, M.D., CHATER, B.V., DUFFIELD, D.P., NEVITT, A.L., O'SULLIVAN, J.J., & STEEL, G.T. (1983) An evaluation of renal function in workers occupationally exposed to mercury vapour. Int. Arch. occup. environ. Health, **52**: 177-189.

STOPFORD, W., BUNDY, S.D., GOLDWATER, L.J., & BIRRIKOFER, K.A. (1978) Microenvironmental exposure to mercury vapor. Am. Ind. Hyg. Assoc. J., **39**: 379-384.

SUGATA, Y. & CLARKSON, T.W. (1979) Exhalation of mercury - further evidence for an oxidation-reduction cycle in mammalian tissues. Biochem. Pharmacol., **28**: 3474-3476.

SUGITA, M. (1978) The biological half-time of heavy metals. The existence of a third "slowest" component. Int. Arch. occup. environ. Health, **41**: 25-40.

SUMMERS, A.O., WIREMAN, J., VIMY, M.J., & LORSCHEIDER, F.L. (1990) Increased mercury resistance in monkey gingival and intestinal bacterial flora after placement of dental "silver" fillings. Physiologist, **33**(4): abstract 116.

SUTER, K. (1975) Studies on the dominant-lethal and fertility effects of the heavy metal compounds methylmercuric hydroxide, mercuric chloride, and cadmium chloride in male and female mice. Mutat. Res., **30**: 363-374.

SUZUKI, T., SHISHIDO, S., & ISHIHARA, N. (1976) Interaction of inorganic to organic mercury in their metabolism in human body. Int. Arch. occup. environ. Health, **38**: 103-113.

SUZUKI, T., TAKEMOTO, T.I., SHISHIDO, S., & KANI, K. (1977) Mercury in human amniotic fluid. Scand. J. Work Environ. Health, **9**: 32-35.

SUZUKI, T., HIMENO, S., HONGO, T., & WATANABE, C. (1986) Mercury-selenium interaction in workers exposed to elemental mercury vapor. J. appl. Toxicol., **6**: 149-153.

SVARE, C.W., PETERSON, L.C., REINHARDT, J.W., BOYER, D.B., FRANK, C.W., GAY, D.D., & COX, R.D. (1981) The effect of dental amalgams on mercury levels in expired air. J. dent. Res., **60**(9): 1668-1671.

SWEDISH ENVIRONMENTAL PROTECTION BOARD (1986) Mercury: occurrence and turnover of mercury in the environment, Stockholm, National Environmental Protection Board, (Mercury Report No. 3).

TAKAHATA, N., HAYASHI, H., WATANABE, S., & ANSO, T. (1970) Accumulation of mercury in the brains of two autopsy cases with chronic inorganic mercury poisoning. Folia psychiatr. neurol. Jpn., **24**(1): 59-69.

TAKIZAWA, Y. (1986) Mercury content in recognized patients and non-recognized patients exposed to methylmercury from Minamata Bay in the last ten years. In: Tsubaki, T. & Takahashi, H., ed. Recent advances in Minamata disease studies, Tokyo, Kodansha Ltd., pp. 24-39.

THOMSON, J. & RUSSELL, J.A. (1970) Dermatitis due to mercury following amalgam dental restorations. Br. J. Dermatol., **82**: 292-297.

TRIEBIG, G. & SCHALLER, K.-H. (1982) Neurotoxic effects in mercury-exposed workers. Neurobehav. Toxicol. Teratol., **4**: 717-720.

TRIEBIG, G., SCHALLER, K.-H., & VALENTIN, H. (1981) [Investigations on neurotoxicity of chemical substances at the workplace. I. Determination of motor and sensory nerve conduction velocity in persons occupationally exposed to mercury.] Int. Arch. occup. environ. Health, **48**: 119-129 (in German with English summary).

TROEN, P., KAUFMAN, S.A., & KATZ, K.H. (1951) Mercuric bichloride poisoning. New Eng. J. Med., **244**(13): 459-463.

TUNNESSEN, W.W., Jr, MCMAHON, K.J., & BASER, M. (1987) Acrodynia: exposure to mercury from fluorescent light bulbs. Pediatrics, **79**(5): 786-789.

UMEDA, M. & NISHIMURA, M. (1979) Inducibility of chromosomal aberrations by metal compounds in cultured mammalian cells. Mutat. Res., **67**: 221-229.

UNEP/WHO (1984) Principles and procedures for quality assurance in environmental pollution: Exposure monitoring, Geneva, World Health Organization (EFP/HEAL/84.4).

US ENVIRONMENTAL PROTECTION AGENCY (1989) Integrated risk information system (IRIS): Mercury (inorganic) file data 9/01/81, Cincinnati, Ohio, US Environmental Protection Agency, Environmental Criteria and Assessment Office.

VAHTER, M. (1982) Assessment of human exposure to lead and cadmium through biological monitoring, Stockholm, National Swedish Institute of Environmental Medicine and Department of Environmental Hygiene, Karolinska Institute, 136 pp. (Prepared for the United Nations Environment Programme and the World Health Organization).

VELASQUEZ, E., HASSAN, A., BELMAR, R., DRUCKER, E., & MICHAELS, D. (1980) Occupational mercury poisoning - Nicaragua. CDC Mortal. Morb. Wkly Rep., **29**: 393-395.

VERBERK, M.M., SALLE, H.J.A., & KEMPER, C.H. (1986) Tremor in workers with low exposure to metallic mercury. Am. Ind. Hyg. Assoc. J., **47**: 559-562.

VERSCHAEVE, L. & SUSANNE, C. (1979) Genetic hazards of mercury exposure in dental surgery. Mutat. Res., **64**: 149.

VERSCHAEVE, L., KIRSCH-VOLDERS, M., SUSANNE, C., GROETENBRIEL, C., HAUSTERMANS, R., LECOMTE, A., & ROOSSELS, D. (1976) Genetic damage induced by occupationally low mercury exposure. Environ. Res., **12**: 303-316.

VERSCHAEVE, L., TASSIGNON, J.-P., LEFEVRE, M., DE STOOP, P., & SUSANNE, C. (1979) Cytogenetic investigation on leucocytes of workers exposed to metallic mercury. Environ. Mutagen., **1**: 259-268.

VERSCHAEVE, I., KIRSCH-VOLDERS, M., & SUSANNE, C. (1984) Mercury-induced segregational errors of chromosomes in human lymphocytes and in Indian muntjac cells. Toxicol. Let., **21**: 247-253.

VERSCHAEVE, I., KIRSCH-VOLDERS, M., HENS, L., & SUSANNE, C. (1985) Comparative in vitro cytogenetic studies in mercury-exposed human lymphocytes. Mutat. Res., 157: 221-226.

VILLALUZ, M.G. (1988) Environmental impact assessment of small scale gold mining operations in Davao del Norte. Quezon City, University of the Philippines, College of Engineering (Thesis).

VIMY, M.J. & LORSCHEIDER, F.L. (1985a) Intra-oral air mercury released from dental amalgam. J. dent. Res., 64(8): 1069-1071.

VIMY, M.J. & LORSCHEIDER, F.L. (1985b) Serial measurements of intra-oral air mercury: Estimation of daily dose from dental amalgam. J. dent. Res., 64(8): 1072-1085.

VIMY, M.J., LUFT, A.J., & LORSCHEIDER, F.L. (1986) Estimation of mercury body burden from dental amalgam: Computer simulation of a metabolic compartmental model. J. dent. Res., 65(12): 1415-1419.

VIMY, M.J., TAKAHASHI, Y., & LORSCHEIDER, F.L. (1990a) Maternal-fetal distribution of mercury (Hg^{203}) released from dental amalgam tooth restorations in sheep. Am. J. Physiol., 258 (in press)

VIMY, M.J., BOYD, N.D., HOOPER, D.E., & LORSCHEIDER, F.L. (1990b) Glomerular filtration impairment by mercury released from dental "silver" fillings in sheep. Physiologist, 33(4): abstract 94.

WAHLBERG, J.E. (1965) "Disappearance measurements", a method for studying percutaneous absorption of isotope-labeled compounds emitting gamma-rays. Acta dermato-venereol., 45: 397-414.

WALLINGFORD, K.M. (1982) Health hazard evaluation report, Cincinnati, Ohio, National Institute for Occupational Safety and Health, 7 pp. (HETA 82-364-1243).

WANDS, J.R., WEISS, S.W., YARDLEY, J.H., & MADDREY, W.C. (1974) Chronic inorganic mercury poisoning due to laxative abuse. A clinical and ultrastructural study. Am. J. Med., 57: 92-101.

WARKANY, J. (1966) Acrodynia - postmorten of a disease. Am. J. Dis. Child., 112: 147-156.

WATANABE, T., SHIMADA, T., & ENDO, A. (1982) Effects of mercury compounds on ovulation and meiotic and mitotic chromosomes in female golden hamster. Teratology, 25: 381-384.

WEENING, J.J., FLEUREN, G.J., & HOEDEMAEKER, Ph.J. (1978) Demonstration of antinuclear antibodies in mercuric chloride-induced glomerulopahty in the rat. Lab. Invest., 39(4): 405-411.

WEENING, J.J., HOEDEMAEKER, J., & BAKKER, W.W. (1981) Immunoregulation and antinuclear antibodies in mercury-induced glomerulopathy in the rat. Clin. exp. Immunol., 45: 64-71.

WESSEL, W. (1967) [Electron microscopic contribution to the acute and chronic mercury bichloride and viomycin poisoning of the kidney.] Verh. Dtsch. Ges. Pathol., 51: 313-316 (In German with English summary).

WHITE, R.R. & BRANDT, R.L. (1976) Development of mercury hypersensitivity among dental students. J. Am. Dent. Assoc., 92: 1204-1207.

WHO (1976) Environmental Health Criteria 1: Mercury, Geneva, World Health Organization, 131 pp.

WHO (1980) Recommended health-based limits in occupational exposure to heavy metals. Report of a WHO Study Group, Geneva, World Health Organization, 116 pp. (WHO Technical Report Series, No. 647).

WHO (1986) Guidelines for integrated air, water, food and biological exposure monitoring, Geneva, World Health Organization, UNEP/WHO Global Environmental Monitoring System, HEAL Project (document PEP/86.6).

WHO (1989) Environmental Health Criteria 86: Mercury - Environmental aspects, Geneva, World Health Organization, 115 pp.

WHO (1990) Environmental Health Criteria 101: Methylmercury, Geneva, World Health Organization, 144 pp.

WOLFF, M., OSBORNE, J.W., & HANSON, A.L. (1983) Mercury toxicity and dental amalgam. Neurotoxicology, 4(3): 201-204.

WU, D.L. (1989) [Atmospheric pollution and mercury poisoning caused by peasants mercury smelting.] Chin. J. prev. Med., 23: 83-86 (in Chinese with summary in English).

YOSHIDA, M. & YAMAMURA, Y. (1982) Elemental mercury in urine from workers exposed to mercury vapour. Int. Arch. occup. environ. Health, 51: 99-104.

YOSHIDA, M., YAMAMURA, Y., & SATOH, H. (1986) Distribution of mercury in guinea-pig offspring after in utero exposure to mercury vapor during late gestation. Arch. Toxicol., 58: 225-228.

YOSHIDA, M., AOYAMA, H., SATOH, H., & YAMAMURA, Y. (1987) Binding of mercury to metallothionein-like protein in fetal liver of the guinea pig following in utero exposure to mercury vapor. Toxicol. Lett., 37: 1-6.

YOSHIDA, M., SATOH, H., KOJIMA, S., & YAMAMURA, Y. (1989) Distribution of mercury in neonatal guinea-pigs after exposure to mercury vapours. Bull. environ. Contam. Toxicol., 43(5): 697-704.

YOSHIKAWA, H. & OHTA, H. (1982) Interaction of metals and metallothionein. In: Foulkes, E.C., ed. Biological roles of metallothionein, Amsterdam, Oxford, New York, Elsevier Science Publishers, pp. 11-23.

ZAMPOLLO, A., BARUFFINI, A., CIRLA, A.M., PISATI, G., & ZEDDA, S. (1987) Subclinical inorganic mercury neuropathy: Neurophysiological investigations in 17 occupationally exposed subjects. Ital. J. neurol. Sci., **8**: 249-254.

ZASUKHINA, G.D., VASILYEVA, I.M., SDIRKOVA, N.I., KRASOVSKY, G.N., VASYUKOVICH, L.Ya., KENESARIEV, U.I., & BUTENKO, P.G. (1983) Mutagenic effect of thallium and mercury salts on rodent cells with different repair activities. Mutat. Res., **124**: 163-173.

ZEGLIO, P. (1958) [Long-term effects of mercurialism]. Lav. Um., X: 420-422 (in Italian).

ZIFF, S. (1984) Silver dental fillings - The toxic time bomb. Can the mercury in your dental fillings poison you? New York, Aurora Press, 150 pp.

RESUME ET CONCLUSIONS

La présente monographie est essentiellement consacrée aux risques pour la santé humaine imputables au mercure minéral; elle passe en revue les résultats des recherches qui ont été publiés depuis la parution des Critères d'hygiène de l'environnement No 1: Mercure (WHO, 1977). Depuis 1977, on dispose de nouvelles données concernant la présence de mercure dans les amalgames dentaires et dans les savons éclaircissants, qui constituent deux importants sujets de préoccupation. Dans la présente monographie on insiste principalement sur l'exposition résultant de ces deux utilisations, mais on étudie également les données cinétiques et toxicologiques fondamentales susceptibles d'être utiles dans l'étude de l'ensemble des effets du mercure minéral.

En ce qui concerne la santé humaine, les problèmes liés au transport, à la bioaccumulation et la transformation du mercure minéral à l'échelon planétaire proviennent presque exclusivement de sa conversion en méthylmercure et de l'exposition ultérieure au méthylmercure par l'intermédiaire des fruits de mer ou autres denrées alimentaires. Les aspects environnementaux et écologiques généraux du mercure minéral sont récapitulés dans la présente monographie. On pourra trouver un exposé plus détaillé de ces questions dans les Critères d'hygiène de l'environnement No 86: Mercure - aspects écologiques (WHO, 1989) ainsi que dans les Critères d'hygiène de l'environnement No 101: Méthylmercure (WHO, 1990).

1. Identité

Le mercure existe aux trois degrés d'oxydation suivants: Hg^0 (mercure métallique); Hg_2^{++} (mercure mercureux) et Hg^{++} (mercure mercurique). Il peut former des dérivés organométalliques dont quelques-uns sont utilisés dans l'industrie et en agriculture.

2. Propriétés physiques et chimiques

Le mercure élémentaire a une très forte tension de vapeur. Dans l'atmosphère saturée à 20 °C, sa concentration est 200 fois plus élevée que celle qui est actuellement admise sur les lieux de travail.

La solubilité dans l'eau augmente selon la séquence: mercure élémentaire < chlorure mercureux < chlorure de méthylmercure < chlorure mercurique. Le mercure élémentaire ainsi que les dérivés halogénés des composés alkylmercuriels sont solubles dans les solvants apolaires.

Les vapeurs de mercure sont plus solubles dans le plasma, le sang total et l'hémoglobine que dans l'eau distillée où la solubilité est très faible. Les dérivés organométalliques sont stables mais certains d'entre eux sont facilement dégradés par les organismes vivants.

3. Méthodes d'analyse

Les méthodes les plus couramment utilisées pour le dosage du mercure total et du mercure minéral sont l'absorption atomique de la vapeur froide (CVAA) et l'activation neutronique. On trouvera un exposé détaillé des méthodes d'analyse dans les Critères d'hygiène de l'environnement No 1: Mercure (WHO, 1977) ainsi que dans le No 101: Méthylmercure (WHO, 1990).

Pour toutes ces méthodes d'analyse, une assurance minutieuse de la qualité est indispensable.

3.1 Analyses, prélèvements et conservation des urines

Pour l'analyse de routine des divers milieux, on a recours à la spectrophotométrie d'absorption atomique sans flamme. Il faut être spécialement prudent lors du choix des anticoagulants utilisés pour les prélèvements sanguins afin d'éviter toute contamination par des dérivés mercuriels. Des précautions particulières sont également nécessaires lors du prélèvement et de la conservation des urines car la croissance bactérienne peut modifier la concentration des nombreuses formes de mercure susceptibles d'être présentes dans les urines. Pour éviter l'altération des échantillons d'urine, la meilleure méthode consiste à les additionner d'acide chlorhydrique ou d'un bactéricide puis de congeler l'échantillon. Il est recommandé de procéder à une correction en concentration relativement à la densité des urines ou à la teneur en créatinine.

3.2 Analyses et échantillonnage de l'air

Le dosage du mercure dans l'air peut s'effectuer soit par des méthodes à lecture instantanée soit par des méthodes qui comportent deux phases distinctes: échantillonnage et analyse. Les méthodes à lecture instantanée peuvent être utilisées pour le dosage des vapeurs de mercure. Pour le dosage du mercure total, l'échantillonnage s'effectue en milieu oxydant acide ou sur hopcalite.

Le dosage par absorption atomique de la vapeur froide (CVAA) est la méthode la plus fréquemment utilisée.

4. Sources d'exposition humaine et environnementale

4.1 Etat naturel

Le mercure présent dans la nature provient principalement du dégazage de la croûte terrestre, des éruptions volcaniques et de l'évaporation des étendues d'eau.

Les émissions d'origine naturelle sont de l'ordre de 2700 à 6000 tonnes par an.

4.2 Sources d'origine humaine

On estime à 10 000 tonnes la quantité de mercure extraite chaque année dans le monde. Cette activité entraîne un certain nombre de pertes dans l'environnement ainsi qu'une décharge directe dans l'atmosphère. Parmi les autres sources importantes de pollution par le mercure, on compte l'utilisation des combustibles fossiles, le grillage des minerais métalliques sulfurés, le raffinage de l'or, la production de ciment, l'incinération des déchets et diverses opérations métallurgiques.

Une installation de production électrolytique de chlore et de soude donne normalement lieu à des émissions de mercure de l'ordre de 450 g par tonne de soude caustique produite.

La quantité totale libérée annuellement dans l'atmosphère de la planète par suite d'activités humaines atteint quelque 3000 tonnes.

5. Usages

Le mercure est principalement utilisé comme cathode dans l'électrolyse du chlorure de sodium. Etant donné que les produits de cette électrolyse sont contaminés par du mercure, leur emploi dans des opérations industrielles ultérieures provoque la contamination d'autres produits. Le mercure est également utilisé dans l'industrie électrique, pour la fabrication d'instruments de mesure utilisés dans les ménages ou dans l'industrie ainsi que pour la fabrication d'instruments de laboratoire et d'appareils médicaux. Certains médicaments contiennent du mercure minéral. On utilise également une très grande quantité de mercure pour l'extraction de l'or.

Les amalgames utilisés en art dentaire pour l'obturation des dents contiennent une grande quantité de mercure mélangée (en proportion de 1:1) avec un alliage pulvérulent à base d'argent, d'étain, de cuivre et de zinc. L'amalgame au cuivre, utilisé essentiellement pour les soins dentaires aux enfants, contient jusqu'à 70% de mercure et jusqu'à 30% de cuivre. Il peut en résulter une exposition du dentiste, de ses assistants et des patients au mercure.

Certaines personnes de couleur utilisent des crèmes et des savons à base de mercure pour s'éclaircir la peau. Ces produits sont désormais interdits dans la Communauté européenne, en Amérique du Nord et dans de nombreux pays d'Afrique mais on fabrique encore des savons à base de mercure dans plusieurs pays d'Europe. Les savons contiennent jusqu'à 3% d'iodure de mercure et les crèmes jusqu'à 10% de mercure ammoniacal.

6. Transport, distribution et transformation dans l'environnement

Le mercure émis dans l'atmosphère sous forme de vapeur est transformé en dérivés solubles et il se dépose avec les précipitations sur le sol et dans l'eau. La vapeur de mercure peut subsister jusqu'à trois ans dans l'atmosphère, cette période étant réduite à quelques semaines dans le cas des formes solubles.

La première étape du processus de bioaccumulation aquatique consiste dans la transformation du mercure minéral en méthylmercure. Cette transformation s'opère soit par voie non enzymatique soit sous l'action de microorganismes. Le méthylmercure pénètre dans la chaîne alimentaire des espèces prédatrices où il subit une bioamplification.

7. Exposition humaine

C'est principalement par l'intermédiaire des aliments et des amalgames dentaires que la population générale est exposée au mercure. En fonction de l'importance de sa concentration dans l'air et dans l'eau, la dose totale ingérée quotidiennement peut s'en trouver notablement augmentée. Le poisson constitue la source principale d'exposition humaine au méthylmercure. Des études expérimentales récentes ont montré que le mercure libéré dans la cavité buccale à partir d'un amalgame l'est sous forme de vapeur. La mastication augmente la vitesse de libération de ces vapeurs. Un certain nombre d'études ont montré qu'il y avait une corrélation entre le nombre d'obturations au moyen d'un amalgame ou de surfaces recouvertes d'amalgame et la teneur en mercure des tissus, mesurée après autopsie, ainsi que la teneur en mercure du sang, des urines et du plasma. L'absorption de mercure calculée à partir de la quantité d'amalgame et l'accumulation effectivement observée présente d'importantes variations individuelles. Il est donc difficile de procéder à des estimations précises de la quantité de mercure provenant des amalgames dentaires qui finit par se fixer dans l'organisme. Des études expérimentales effectuées sur des moutons ont permis d'étudier plus en détail la distribution du mercure provenant des amalgames dentaires.

L'utilisation de savons et de crèmes pour s'éclaircir la peau peut également donner lieu à une importante exposition.

On a étudié l'exposition professionnelle au mercure minéral dans les unités d'électrolyse du chlorure de sodium, dans les mines de mercure, les fabriques de thermomètres, les raffineries et les cabinets dentaires. Pour tous ces types d'exposition professionnelle, on a relevé d'importantes quantités de mercure, mais celles-ci varient en fonction des ambiances de travail.

8. Cinétique et métabolisme

Les études sur l'homme et l'animal montrent qu'après inhalation de vapeur de mercure, la proportion retenue par l'organisme est d'environ 80% alors qu'elle est inférieure à 1% lorsque le mercure métallique est ingéré sous forme liquide, ce qui témoigne d'une faible absorption dans les voies digestives. Après inhalation, les aérosols de mercure minéral se déposent dans les voies respiratoires et sont absorbés à une vitesse qui dépend de la taille des particules. Il est probable que les composés minéraux du mercure sont absorbés dans les voies digestives dans une proportion qui est en moyenne inférieure à 10%, mais là encore les variations individuelles sont considérables. L'absorption est beaucoup plus élevée chez les ratons nouveau-nés.

C'est principalement au niveau des reins que se dépose le mercure après administration de vapeur de mercure élémentaire ou de dérivés minéraux du mercure (cela représente 50 à 90% de la charge totale de l'organisme chez l'animal). Après inhalation de mercure élémentaire on observe que la quantité de mercure qui passe dans le cerveau, chez des souris et des singes, est nettement plus élevée qu'après injection intraveineuse équivalente sous forme de sels mercuriques. Chez l'homme, le rapport hématies/plasma est plus élevé ($>$ 1) après administration de mercure élémentaire qu'après administration d'un sel mercurique et la quantité de mercure qui traverse la barrière placentaire est plus importante. Seule une faible fraction de la quantité de mercure administrée sous forme de sels bivalents pénètre dans l'organisme du foetus de rat.

Plusieurs types de transformation métabolique peuvent se produire:

• oxydation du mercure métallique en mercure (II);
• réduction du mercure (II) en mercure métallique;
• méthylation du mercure minéral;
• conversion du méthylmercure en mercure minéral bivalent.

L'oxydation des vapeurs de mercure métallique en mercure ionique bivalent (section 6.1.1) n'est pas suffisamment rapide pour empêcher le passage du mercure élémentaire à travers la barrière hémo-méningée, à travers le placenta ou d'autres tissus. Dans ces tissus, l'oxydation piège le mercure qui s'accumule dans le cerveau et les tissus du foetus.

La réduction du mercure (II) en mercure (0) a été observée tant chez l'animal (rats et souris) que chez l'homme. Inversement, la décomposition d'organomercuriels tels que le méthylmercure constitue une source de mercure (II).

C'est principalement par la voie fécale et par la voie urinaire que s'élimine chez l'homme le mercure minéral encore qu'il puisse être exhalé en petites quantités sous forme élémentaire. Il peut également se produire une déplétion tissulaire par transfert des tissus maternels à ceux du foetus.

La demi-vie biologique, qui pour la majeure partie du mercure s'étend de quelques jours à quelques semaines, peut être très longue - jusqu'à plusieurs années - pour la fraction restante. Ces demi-vies très longues ont été observées tant chez l'animal que chez l'homme. Il se produit une interaction complexe entre le mercure et certains autres éléments, notamment le sélénium. Il se pourrait que la très longue demi-vie d'élimination d'une fraction du mercure s'explique par la formation d'un complexe avec le sélénium.

8.1 Valeurs de référence et valeurs normales

Les quelques données dont on dispose à propos de mineurs décédés montrent que plusieurs années après l'arrêt de l'exposition, la concentration du mercure dans le cerveau était encore de plusieurs mg/kg, avec des valeurs encore plus élevées dans certaines zones. Toutefois cette analyse n'ayant pas fait l'objet d'un contrôle de qualité, les données demeurent incertaines. Chez un petit nombre de dentistes examinés après leur mort et qui ne présentaient pas de symptômes d'hydrargyrisme, on a observé que les teneurs en mercure allaient de très faibles concentrations jusqu'à des valeurs de quelques centaines de μg/kg dans le cortex du lobe occipital et d'environ 100 μg/kg à quelques mg/kg dans l'hypophyse.

L'examen post-mortem de sujets qui n'étaient pas professionnellement exposés au mercure mais étaient porteurs d'un certain nombre d'obturations au moyen d'amalgame, a montré qu'un nombre modéré (environ 25) de surfaces recouvertes d'amalgame augmentent en moyenne la concentration cérébrale du mercure d'à peu près 10 μg/kg. L'augmentation correspondante au niveau des reins, déterminée au moyen d'un nombre très limité d'analyses est probablement de 300 à 400 μg/kg. Toutefois les variations individuelles sont considérables.

La concentration du mercure dans les urines et le sang peut être utilisée comme indicateur de l'exposition, à condition que celle-ci soit relativement constante, qu'elle soit prolongée et déterminée sur un groupe de sujets. Les données récentes sont plus fiables que celles dont il est fait état dans les Critères d'hygiène de l'environnement No 1: Mercure (WHO, 1977). Après exposition professionnelle à des quantités de mercure d'environ 40 μg/m^3 d'air, on observe des concentrations urinaires d'environ 50 μg/g de créatinine. Ce rapport (5:4) entre les concentrations urinaires et les concentrations atmosphériques est beaucoup plus faible que le rapport de 3:1 auquel étaient parvenus les experts de WHO (1977). La différence peut s'expliquer en partie par des variations dans les techniques d'échantillonnage utilisées pour calculer l'exposition atmosphérique. Une exposition de l'ordre de 40 μg/m^3 d'air correspond à environ 15-20 μg de mercure par litre de sang. Toutefois, il peut être difficile d'évaluer l'exposition à de faibles concentrations de mercure inorganique par analyse du sang lorsqu'il y a exposition simultanée au méthylmercure. Pour lever la difficulté, on peut procéder au dosage du mercure dans le plasma ou doser simultanément le mercure minéral et le méthylmercure. Le méthylmercure est beaucoup moins gênant lorsqu'on procède à une analyse d'urine car il n'est excrété dans les urines qu'en très faible proportion.

9. Effets chez l'homme

Une exposition aiguë au mercure par inhalation de vapeurs peut occasionner des douleurs thoraciques, de la dyspnée, de la toux, une hémoptysie et quelquefois provoquer une pneumonie interstitielle mortelle. L'ingestion de dérivés mercuriques, en particulier de chlorure mercurique, peut provoquer une gastro-entérite ulcérative et une nécrose tubulaire aiguë suspectible d'entraîner la mort par anurie si l'on ne dispose pas de moyens de dialyse.

En cas d'exposition aux vapeurs de mercure, c'est le système nerveux central qui constitue l'organe critique. L'exposition subaiguë peut entraîner des réactions psychotiques caractérisées par un délire, des hallucinations et une tendance suicidaire. L'exposition professionnelle peut conduire à des troubles fonctionnels très variés dont l'éréthisme constitue la caractéristique essentielle. Lorsque l'exposition se poursuit, on voit apparaître de légers tremblements, initialement au niveau des mains. Dans les cas bénins d'éréthisme, ces tremblements régressent lentement en quelques années après cessation de l'exposition. On a constaté chez des travailleurs exposés au mercure une diminution de la vitesse de conduction nerveuse. Des symptômes d'éréthisme moins prononcés ont été observés à la suite d'une exposition prolongée à de faibles concentrations.

On connaît très mal les concentrations de mercure dans le cerveau dans les cas d'hydrargyrisme et on ne peut pas évaluer la dose sans effet observable ni tracer une courbe dose-réponse.

Lorsque le taux d'excrétion urinaire du mercure atteint 100 μg/g de créatinine, il existe une forte probabilité pour qu'apparaissent les signes neurologiques classiques de l'hydraargyrisme (tremblements, éréthisme) et l'on note une forte protéinurie. Une exposition de 30 à 100 μg de mercure/g de créatinine entraîne une incidence accrue de certains effets toxiques de moindre gravité qui ne se traduisent pas par une détérioration clinique manifeste. Dans quelques études, on a observé des tremblements, enregistrés par voie électrophysiologique, à des concentrations faibles dans l'urine (pouvant s'abaisser jusqu'à 25-35 μg/g de créatinine). En revanche, d'autres études n'ont pas mis cet effet en évidence. Certaines des personnes exposées font une protéinurie (protéines de faibles masse moléculaire relative et micro-albuminurie). On ne dispose pas de données épidémiologiques appropriées pour les taux d'exposition qui correspondent à moins de 30-50 μg de mercure/g de créatinine.

L'exposition de la population générale est en principe faible mais dans certains cas, elle peut atteindre les valeurs constatées dans les ambiances de travail et même conduire à des intoxications. C'est ainsi que des erreurs de manipulation de mercure liquide ont pu conduire à de graves intoxications.

Après ingestion de sels de mercure bivalent, c'est le rein, qui est l'organe critique. On sait depuis longtemps que l'exposition professionnelle au mercure métallique entraîne une protéinurie tant chez les travailleurs présentant des signes d'hydrargyrisme que chez ceux qui sont asymptomatiques. On observe moins fréquemment un syndrome néphrotique, syndrome qui peut également se produire après utilisation de crèmes à base de mercure pour s'éclaircir la peau et même après une exposition accidentelle. Il semblerait d'après les données actuelles que ce syndrome néphrotique soit dû à une réaction immunotoxique. Jusqu'à ces derniers temps, on n'avait signalé d'effets néphrotoxiques de la vapeur de mercure qu'à des doses supérieures à celles qui entraînent l'apparition de symptômes centraux. Cependant des études nouvelles font état d'effets rénaux à des concentrations plus faibles. L'expérimentation animale montre que le mercure minéral peut provoquer une glomérulonéphrite auto-immune. Cet effet s'observe chez toutes les espèces à l'exception de certaines souches, ce qui indique l'existence d'une prédisposition génétique. Une étiologie immunologique a pour conséquence, en l'absence d'études dose-réponse sur des groupes d'individus immunologiquement réceptifs, l'impossibilité d'établir scientifiquement la dose limite de mercure (par exemple dans le sang ou les urines) en dessous de laquelle (dans les cas individuels) il n'y aura pas de symptômes d'hydrargyrisme.

Les vapeurs de mercure et les dérivés mercuriels peuvent provoquer des dermatites de contact. Des produits pharmaceutiques à base de mercure ont provoqué des cas d'acrodynie infantile et on tient l'exposition aux vapeurs de mercure pour responsable de la maladie de "Kawasaki". Certaines études, contrairement à d'autres, ont mis en évidence des effets sur le cycle menstruel et sur le développement foetal. Il ressort des études épidémiologiques qui ont été publiées qu'il n'y a pour l'instant pas de réponse à la question de savoir si, en l'absence des signes bien connus de l'intoxication mercurielle, la vapeur de mercure peut avoir des effets nocifs sur le cycle menstruel ou le développement foetal.

Récemment, on a beaucoup débattu de la sécurité des amalgames utilisés en art dentaire et certains ont avancé que l'emploi d'amalgames à base de mercure comportait de graves dangers pour la santé. Les rapports qui font état de différents types de symptômes, de même que les résultats des quelques études épidémiologiques qui ont été effectuées, ne sont pas concluants.

RESUMEN Y CONCLUSIONES

La presente monografía se centra principalmente en el riesgo que representa el mercurio inorgánico para la salud humana y en ella se examinan los informes de investigación aparecidos desde la publicación de Criterios de Salud Ambiental 1: Mercurio (WHO, 1976) (versión española publicada en 1978). Desde 1976, han ido apareciendo nuevos datos de investigación sobre dos importantes cuestiones de salud relacionadas con el mercurio inorgánico, a saber, el mercurio presente en la amalgama de uso odontológico y en los jabones destinados a aclarar la piel. La presente monografía se centra en la exposición a esas dos fuentes, pero se examinan los aspectos cinéticos y toxicológicos elementales teniendo presentes todos los aspectos del mercurio inorgánico.

Los efectos sobre la salud humana relacionados con el transporte mundial, la bioacumulación y la transformación del mercurio inorgánico se derivan casi exclusivamente de la conversión de los compuestos de mercurio en metilmercurio y de la exposición al metilmercurio en los alimentos de origen marino y otros alimentos. En la presente monografía se han resumido los aspectos ambientales y ecológicos mundiales del mercurio inorgánico. Pueden encontrarse descripciones más detalladas en Criterios de Salud Ambiental 86: Mercurio - Aspectos Ambientales (WHO, 1989) y Criterios de Salud Ambiental 101: Metilmercurio (WHO, 1990).

1. Identificación

El mercurio existe en tres estados: Hg^0 (metálico); Hg_2^{++} (mercurioso); y Hg^{++} (mercúrico). Puede formar compuestos organometálicos, algunos de los cuales tienen usos industriales y agrícolas.

2. Propiedades físicas y químicas

El mercurio elemental tiene una presión de vapor sumamente elevada. La atmósfera saturada a 20 °C tiene una concentración más de 200 veces superior a la de la concentración comúnmente aceptada para la exposición profesional.

La solubilidad en el agua aumenta en el orden siguiente: mercurio elemental < cloruro mercurioso < cloruro de metilmercurio < cloruro mercúrico. El mercurio elemental y los haluros de compuestos alquilmercuriales son solubles en disolventes no polares.

El vapor de mercurio es más soluble en plasma, sangre entera y hemoglobina que en agua destilada, donde sólo se disuelve ligeramente. Los compuestos organometálicos son estables, aunque algunos son fácilmente descompuestos por los organismos vivos.

3. Métodos analíticos

Los métodos analíticos más utilizados para cuantificar los compuestos de mercurio total e inorgánico son la absorción atómica sobre vapor frío (AAVF) y la activación de neutrones. Puede encontrarse información detallada sobre los métodos analíticos en Criterios de Salud Ambiental 1: Mercurio (WHO, 1978) y en Criterios de Salud Ambiental 101: Metilmercurio (WHO, 1990).

Todo análisis del mercurio requiere una rigurosa garantía de calidad.

3.1 Análisis, muestreo y conservación de la orina

La espectrofotometría de absorción atómica sin llama se utiliza en los análisis ordinarios para los diversos medios. Debe tenerse especial cuidado al elegir el anticoagulante para el muestreo de sangre a fin de evitar la contaminación por compuestos de mercurio. También debe procederse con suma precaución en el muestreo y el almacenamiento de la orina, puesto que el crecimiento bacteriano es capaz de modificar la concentración de las numerosas formas de mercurio que pueden estar presentes. La adición de ácido clorhídrico o sustancias bactericidas y la congelación son los mejores métodos para impedir la alteración de las muestras de orina. Se recomienda corregir la concentración por referencia a la densidad de la orina o al contenido de creatinina.

3.2 Análisis y muestreo del aire

Los métodos analíticos del mercurio en el aire pueden dividirse en métodos de lectura inmediata y métodos con etapas separadas de muestreo y análisis. Los métodos de lectura inmediata pueden utilizarse para cuantificar el vapor de mercurio elemental. El muestreo en medios acidoxidantes o con hopcalita se usan para cuantificar el mercurio total.

La técnica (AAVF) es el método analítico más frecuente.

4. Fuentes de exposición humana y medioambiental

4.1 Fuentes naturales

Las principales fuentes naturales del mercurio son la desgasificación de la corteza terrestre, las emisiones volcánicas y la evaporación de las masas acuáticas naturales.

Las emisiones naturales son del orden de 2700-6000 toneladas al año.

4.2 Fuentes debidas a la actividad humana

Se estima que la extracción minera del mercurio produce en todo el mundo alrededor de 10 000 toneladas/año. Estas actividades originan ciertas pérdidas de mercurio y descargas directas a la atmósfera. Otras fuentes importantes son la utilización de combustibles fósiles, la fundición de metales con minerales de sulfuro, el refinado del oro, la producción de cemento, la incineración de desechos y las aplicaciones industriales de los metales.

La emisión normal específica de las industrias de compuestos alcalinos del cloro es de aproximadamente 450 g de mercurio por tonelada de sosa cáustica producida.

La cantidad y descarga mundial total de mercurio en la atmósfera debida a las actividades humanas representa hasta 3000 toneladas/año.

5. Usos

Uno de los principales usos del mercurio es como cátodo en la electrólisis del cloruro sódico. Como los compuestos químicos resultantes quedan contaminados con mercurio, su utilización en otras actividades industriales origina la contaminación de otros productos. El mercurio se emplea en la industria eléctrica, en instrumentos de control en el hogar y la industria, y en instrumental médico y de laboratorio. Algunos agentes terapéuticos contienen mercurio inorgánico. En la extracción de oro se utilizan grandes cantidades de mercurio.

La amalgama odontológica de plata para la obturación de dientes contiene grandes cantidades de mercurio, mezclado (en la proporción 1:1) con polvo de aleación (plata, estaño, cobre, zinc). La amalgama de cobre, que se utiliza sobre todo en odontología pediátrica, contiene hasta el 70% de mercurio y hasta el 30% de cobre. Estos usos pueden causar la exposición del dentista, los ayudantes y también de los pacientes.

Algunas personas de piel oscura utilizan cremas y jabones que contienen mercurio para conseguir un tono de piel más claro. La distribución de esos productos está actualmente prohibida en la CEE, en América del Norte y en muchos países africanos, pero en varios países europeos se sigue fabricando jabón con mercurio. Estos jabones contienen hasta un 3% de yoduro de mercurio y las cremas contienen mercurio amoniacal (hasta el 10%).

6. Transporte, distribución y transformación en el medio ambiente

El vapor de mercurio emitido se convierte en formas solubles que son depositadas por la lluvia en el suelo y el agua. El tiempo de persistencia atmosférica para el vapor de mercurio es de hasta tres años, mientras que el de las formas solubles es de sólo algunas semanas.

El cambio de especiación del mercurio desde las formas inorgánicas hasta las metiladas es la primera etapa del proceso de bioacumulación acuática. Esto puede suceder sin el concurso de enzimas o mediante la acción microbiana. El metilmercurio ingresa en la cadena alimentaria de las especies predadoras en las que se produce biomagnificación.

7. Exposición humana

La población general está principalmente expuesta al mercurio por la dieta y la amalgama odontológica.

Atendiendo a las concentraciones en la atmósfera y en el agua, pueden producirse contribuciones importantes a la ingesta diaria de mercurio total. El pescado es una de las fuentes principales de exposición humana al metilmercurio. En estudios experimentales recientes se ha demostrado que el mercurio se libera en forma de vapor desde las restauraciones con amalgama en la boca. La tasa de liberación de este vapor de mercurio aumenta, por ejemplo, al masticar. Varios estudios han correlacionado el número de obturaciones con amalgama odontológica o de superficies de amalgama con el contenido de mercurio en tejidos obtenidos en la autopsia humana, así como en muestras de sangre, orina y plasma. Tanto la ingesta prevista de mercurio a partir de la amalgama como la acumulación observada de mercurio demuestran importantes variaciones individuales. Así pues, resulta difícil cuantificar con exactitud la liberación y la ingestión de mercurio por el cuerpo humano a partir de las restauraciones odontológicas con amalgama. Los estudios experimentales realizados en ovejas han examinado con mayor detalle la distribución del mercurio liberado de las restauraciones con amalgama.

El uso de jabón y cremas para aclarar la piel puede ser origen de una importante exposición al mercurio.

La exposición profesional al mercurio inorgánico se ha estudiado en plantas industriales de productos cloralcalinos, minas de mercurio, fábricas de termómetros, refinerías y consultorios odontológicos. Se han comunicado elevados niveles de mercurio respecto de todas estas situaciones de exposición profesional, si bien los niveles varían en virtud de las condiciones del entorno laboral.

8. Cinética y metabolismo

Los resultados de los estudios realizados tanto en personas como en animales indican que alrededor del 80% del vapor de mercurio metálico inhalado es retenido por el organismo, mientras que el mercurio metálico líquido se absorbe mal en el tracto gastrointestinal (menos del 1%). Los aerosoles de mercurio inorgánico inhalados se depositan en el tracto respiratorio y son absorbidos a una velocidad que depende del tamaño de las partículas. Los compuestos de mercurio inorgánico probablemente son absorbidos desde el tracto gastrointestinal humano hasta un nivel inferior al 10%, en promedio, pero la variación individual es considerable. La absorción es mucho más elevada en la rata recién nacida.

El riñón es el depósito principal de mercurio tras la administración de vapor de mercurio elemental o de compuestos de mercurio inorgánico (50-90% de la carga corporal de los animales). De modo significativo, más mercurio es transportado al cerebro del ratón y el mono tras la inhalación de mercurio elemental que tras la inyección intravenosa de dosis equivalentes de la forma mercúrica. El cociente hematíes:plasma en el hombre es mayor ($\geq$ 1) tras la administración de mercurio elemental que tras la de mercurio mercúrico, y la proporción de mercurio que atraviesa la barrera placentaria es mayor. Sólo una pequeña fracción del mercurio bivalente administrado ingresa en el feto de la rata.

Pueden producirse varias formas de transformación metabólica:

• oxidación del mercurio metálico a mercurio bivalente;
• reducción del mercurio bivalente a mercurio metálico;
• metilación del mercurio inorgánico;
• conversión del metilmercurio en mercurio inorgánico bivalente.

La oxidación de vapor de mercurio metálico a mercurio iónico bivalente (sección 6.1.1) no es lo bastante rápida como para impedir el paso de mercurio elemental a través de la barrera hematoencefálica, la placenta y otros tejidos. La oxidación en esos tejidos sirve como filtro para retener el mercurio y lleva a su acumulación en el cerebro y los tejidos fetales.

La reducción del mercurio bivalente a Hg^0 se ha demostrado tanto en animales (ratones y ratas) como en el hombre. La descomposición de los compuestos organomercuriales, incluido el metilmercurio, es también una fuente de mercurio mercúrico.

Las rutas fecal y urinaria son las principales vías de eliminación del mercurio inorgánico en el hombre, si bien se exhala una pequeña cantidad de mercurio elemental. Una forma de eliminación de mercurio es la transferencia del mercurio materno al feto.

La semivida biológica, que dura sólo unos cuantos días o semanas para la mayor parte del mercurio absorbido, es sumamente larga, probablemente de años, para una parte del mercurio. Esas largas semividas se han observado en experimentos realizados con animales así como en el hombre. Existe una complicada interacción entre el mercurio y algunos elementos, incluido el selenio. La formación de un complejo con el selenio puede ser responsable de la larga semivida que tiene una parte del mercurio.

8.1 Valores de referencia y normales

La limitada información de que se dispone sobre mineros fallecidos muestra la existencia de concentraciones de mercurio en el cerebro de varios mg/kg, años después de finalizar la exposición, con valores aún más altos en algunas partes del cerebro. No obstante, la falta de control de la calidad en el análisis hace inciertos estos datos. Entre un pequeño número de dentistas fallecidos, sin síntomas conocidos de intoxicación por mercurio, los niveles de éste variaron desde concentraciones muy bajas hasta varios cientos de μg/kg en la corteza del lóbulo occipital y desde unos 100 μg/kg hasta unos cuantos mg/kg en la hipófisis.

De las autopsias realizadas en sujetos no expuestos profesionalmente pero con un número variable de obturaciones con amalgama, se desprende que un número moderado (alrededor de 25) de superficies de amalgama pueden, en promedio, aumentar la concentración de mercurio en el cerebro en unos 10 μg/kg. El aumento correspondiente en el riñón, basado en un número muy limitado de análisis, es probablemente de 300-400 μg/kg. Sin embargo, la variación individual es considerable.

Los niveles de mercurio en la orina y la sangre pueden usarse como indicadores de la exposición, siempre que ésta sea relativamente constante a largo plazo y se evalúe en un grupo. Los datos de exposición recientes son más fiables que los que se citan en Criterios de Salud Ambiental 1: Mercurio (WHO, 1978). Se observan niveles en la orina de unos 50 μg/g de creatinina tras la exposición profesional a unos 40 μg de mercurio por m^3 de aire. Esta relación (5:4) entre orina y niveles atmosféricos es mucho más baja que la de 3:1 estimada por la WHO (1976).

La diferencia puede deberse en parte a la distinta técnica de muestreo para evaluar la exposición atmosférica. Una exposición de 40 μg de mercurio/m^3 de aire corresponderá a unos 15-20 μg de mercurio/litro de sangre. Sin embargo, la interferencia debida a la exposición al metilmercurio puede hacer más difícil evaluar la exposición a bajas concentraciones de mercurio inorgánico por medio de análisis de sangre. Una forma de salvar esos problemas es analizar el mercurio en el plasma o analizar tanto el mercurio inorgánico como el metilmercurio. El problema de la interferencia debida al metilmercurio es mucho menor cuando se analiza la orina, puesto que el metilmercurio se excreta con la orina en grado sumamente reducido.

9. Efectos en el hombre

La exposición aguda por inhalación de vapores de mercurio puede verse seguida por dolores de pecho, disnea, tos, hemoptisis, y a veces pneumonitis intersticial que puede provocar la muerte. La ingestión de compuestos mercúricos, en particular cloruro mercúrico, ha provocado casos de gastroenteritis ulcerativa y necrosis tubular aguda, con muerte por anuria en los casos en que no se dispuso de diálisis.

El sistema nervioso central es el órgano crítico para la exposición al vapor de mercurio. La exposición subaguda ha dado origen a reacciones psicóticas caracterizadas por delirio, alucinaciones y tendencias suicidas. La exposición profesional origina eretismo como principal característica de un trastorno funcional de amplio espectro. Si prosigue la exposición, se presenta un temblor fino, que al principio afecta a las manos. En los casos más leves el eretismo y el temblor desaparecen poco a poco a lo largo de varios años, una vez interrumpida la exposición. Se ha demostrado en trabajadores expuestos al mercurio una menor velocidad de conducción nerviosa. La exposición a bajos niveles durante periodos largos se ha asociado a síntomas de eretismo menos pronunciados.

Se dispone de muy poca información sobre los niveles cerebrales de mercurio en los casos de envenenamiento, y no se sabe nada que permita estimar una concentración carente de efectos observados o una curva dosis-respuesta.

Cuando el nivel de excreción urinaria de mercurio es de 100 µg/g de creatinina, hay una probabilidad muy alta de que aparezcan los signos neurológicos clásicos de la intoxicación por mercurio (temblor, eretismo) y proteinuria. Una exposición correspondiente a 30 hasta 100 µg de mercurio/g de creatinina aumenta la incidencia de algunos efectos tóxicos menos graves que no provocan trastornos clínicos manifiestos. En algunos estudios se han observado temblores, electrofisiológicamente registrados, a concentraciones urinarias reducidas (tan bajas como 25-35 µg/g de creatinina). En otros estudios no se observó ese efecto. Algunas de las personas expuestas presentan proteinuria (proteínas de baja masa molecular relativa y microalbuminuria). No se dispone de datos epidemiológicos adecuados sobre los niveles de exposición que corresponden a menos de 30-50 µg de mercurio/g de creatinina.

Aunque la exposición de la población general es por lo general reducida, en ocasiones puede elevarse hasta el nivel de exposición profesional y puede incluso llegar a ser tóxica. Así, la manipulación incorrecta de mercurio líquido ha dado origen a casos graves de intoxicación.

El riñón es el órgano crítico tras la ingestión de sales de mercurio bivalente inorgánico. La exposición profesional a mercurio metálico se asocia desde hace tiempo a la aparición de proteinuria, tanto en obreros con otros síntomas de envenenamiento por mercurio como en aquéllos sin esos síntomas. En otros casos menos frecuentes, la exposición profesional se ha visto seguida del síndrome nefrótico, que también se ha producido tras el uso de cremas para aclarar la piel con mercurio inorgánico, e incluso tras la exposición accidental. Las pruebas actuales sugieren que este síndrome nefrótico se debe a una respuesta inmunotóxica. Hasta hace poco, los efectos del vapor de mercurio elemental en el riñón se habían comunicado sólo con respecto a dosis más elevadas que las asociadas a la aparición de signos y síntomas del sistema nervioso central. En los nuevos estudios, no obstante, se han notificado efectos en el riñón con niveles inferiores de exposición. Los estudios experimentales con animales han demostrado que el mercurio puede inducir glomerulonefritis autoinmune en todas las especies ensayadas, pero no en todas las estirpes, lo que indica una predisposición genética. Una de las consecuencias de la etiología inmunológica es que, en ausencia de estudios de la dosis-respuesta en grupos de individuos inmunológicamente sensibles, resulta científicamente imposible establecer un nivel de mercurio (por ejemplo, en la sangre o la orina) por debajo del cual (en casos individuales) no se producirán síntomas relacionados con el mercurio.

Tanto los vapores de mercurio metálico como los compuestos de mercurio han dado origen a dermatitis de contacto. Los productos farmacéuticos con mercurio han sido responsables de la "enfermedad rosada" en los niños, y la exposición al vapor de mercurio ha sido responsable de la enfermedad de "Kawasaki". En algunos estudios, pero no en todos, se han comunicado efectos en el ciclo menstrual y/o en el desarrollo del feto. El nivel de los estudios epidemiológicos publicados aún no permite saber si los vapores de mercurio pueden afectar negativamente al ciclo menstrual o al desarrollo del feto sin que se observen los conocidos síntomas de la intoxicación por mercurio.

Hace poco ha habido una intensa polémica sobre la inocuidad de las amalgamas odontológicas y se ha afirmado que el mercurio de la amalgama puede plantear graves peligros para la salud. Los informes en los que se describen distintos tipos de síntomas y signos y los resultados de los escasos estudios epidemiológicos realizados no son concluyentes.

www.ingramcontent.com/pod-product-compliance
Lightning Source LLC
Chambersburg PA
CBHW071642210326
41597CB00017B/2082